Loudell F. Snow
MSU - 1977

LABOR

AMONG

PRIMITIVE PEOPLES

AMS PRESS
NEW YORK

LABOR

AMONG

PRIMITIVE PEOPLES.

SHOWING

THE DEVELOPMENT OF THE OBSTETRIC SCIENCE OF TO-DAY,

FROM THE

NATURAL AND INSTINCTIVE CUSTOMS

OF

ALL RACES,

CIVILIZED AND SAVAGE, PAST AND PRESENT.

By GEO. J. ENGELMANN, A.M., M.D.

Professor of Obstetrics in the Post-Graduate School of the Missouri Medical College.
Master in Obstetrics of the University of Vienna. Fellow of the American
Gynecological Society; of the London Obstetric Society; of the
Pathological Society of London Consulting Surgeon to
the St. Louis Female Hospital; St. Ann's Lying-in
Asylum; Mexico Hospital, etc.

FIFTY - SIX ILLUSTRATIONS.

ST. LOUIS:
J. H. CHAMBERS & CO.
1882.

Library of Congress Cataloging in Publication Data

Engelmann, George Julius, 1847-1903.
 Labor among primitive peoples, showing the development
of the obstetric science of to-day, from the natural and
instinctive customs of all races, civilized and savage,
past and present.
 Reprint of the 1882 ed. published by J. H. Chambers,
St. Louis.
  1. Obstetrics—History. 2. Labor (Obstetrics)
3. Birth (in religion, folk-lore, etc.) I. Title:
Labor among primitive peoples . . .
RG511.E57   1977   618.2'009   75-23705
ISBN 0-404-13257-X

Reprinted from an original copy in the collections
of the Ohio State University Libraries

From the edition of 1882, St. Louis
First AMS edition published in 1977
Manufactured in the United States of America

AMS PRESS INC.
NEW YORK, N.Y.

INDEX.

CHAPTER I.

POSTURE IN LABOR.

	PAGE
INTRODUCTION.	1
Origin of this paper	1
History of the subject.	2
Plan of the investigation.	4
Division of the subject	6
Assistance received in the work	7
GEOGRAPHICAL DISTRIBUTION OF THE VARIOUS POSITIONS	8

PART I.

	PAGE
POSITION OF PARTURIENT WOMEN AMONG PEOPLES WHOSE LABOR IS GOVERNED BY INSTINCT, AND NOT BY MODERN OBSTETRIC FASHION..	11
A—Perpendicular or upright posture	11
1. Standing	11
2. Partially suspended	14
3. Suspended	18
B—Inclined position	20
1. Sitting erect	20
2. Squatting, as in defecation	22
3. Kneeling.	28
a—The body inclined forward.	29
b—Knee-hand or knee-elbow position.	39
c—The body erect, inclined backward or partially suspended	43
d—Kneeling postures where precise descriptions are lacking	49
4. Semi-recumbent	50
a—Sitting, semi-recumbent on the ground, upon a stone or stool	51
b—Sitting on the lap or between the thighs of an assistant, who is seated on a chair or on the floor	57
c—The obstetric chair	66
d—Semi-recumbent position, strictly speaking	73

                                                                    PAGE
C—Horizontal or recumbent... 78
   1. The dorsal decubitus.. 78
   2. The lateral decubitus... 82
   3. Prone upon the stomach... 83

PART II.

THE POSITION OF WOMEN AMONG CIVILIZED RACES OF THE PRESENT
   DAY IN THE AGONY OF THE EXPULSIVE PAINS............................ 84
RESUME AND CONCLUSIONS... 88
   Résumé 88
   Conclusions... 92

CHAPTER II.

THE THIRD STAGE OF LABOR.

INTRODUCTION 96
MANAGEMENT OF SIMPLE CASES.. 98
   Placenta delivered in the same position which has been occupied dur-
    ing labor-pains and the expulsion of the child.................................
     Manual expression... 98
     Intra-abdominal pressure... 102
     Traction on the cord. 103
   Delivery of the placenta with the patient in a different position from
    the one occupied during the expulsion of the child 104
MANAGEMENT OF THE PLACENTA IN CASE OF RETARDED EXPULSION... 107
MANAGEMENT OF THE UMBILICAL CORD.. 110
PECULIAR SUPERSTITIONS AND CUSTOMS... 112
CONCLUSIONS... 113

CHAPTER III.

PREGNANCY, PARTURITION AND CHILDBED.

PREGNANCY.. 116
PARTURITION 121
   Comparison of labor among civilized and savage races......................... 121
   Accidents in labor among primitive people. 124
   Superstitions and customs... 125
   Place of confinement. 126
   Couch.. 128
   Assistants, midwives, etc 129

PAGE
Kind of assistance rendered.. 131
    Expression... 132
    Fright... 133
    Medicines, herbs... 134
CHILDBED.. 136
    Treatment of the mother..
        Treatment immediately after delivery.......................... 137
        The binder.. 139
        Time of rest accorded... 139
        Diet of the lying-in woman..................................... 143
        Medicines used.. 144
    Management of the child.. 146
        The bath.. 147
        Time of applying the child to the breast................... 148
        Period of nursing... 149
        Weaning.. 149
        Food given in addition to the breast......................... 149
        Medicines used... 151

CHAPTER IV.

MASSAGE AND EXPRESSION.

REVIEW OF THE SUBJECT... 152
A—HISTORY OF MASSAGE... 153
    Ancient times.. 153
    Middle ages.. 154
    Various manipulations practiced.. 154
    Physiological effects.. 155
B—HISTORY OF EXTERNAL MANIPULATIONS IN OBSTETRIC PRACTICE.... 156
    Only help in difficult labor.. 156
    Saying of Hippocrates.. 156
    Greece and Rome... 156
    Savage races of the present... 158
C—THE VARIOUS KINDS OF EXTERNAL MANIPULATIONS...................... 159
    I. Pressure:
        1. By the arms of an assistant encircling the patient's ab-
            domen.. 159
        2. Bandage tightened by assistants...................................... 161
        3. Drawing the abdomen across a rope or pole..................... 163
        4. Stripping down the abdomen.. 164
        5. Expression by means of the feet....................................... 165
        6. The belt.. 165
        7. Pressure against a staff... 166
        8. Lying prone upon the stomach.. 166

PAGE

II. Massage 167
III. Shaking up of the Patient.. 170
IV. Permanent Pressure... 170
D—THE USES OF MASSAGE AND EXPRESSION 171
    I. In pregnancy... 171
        1. Correcting malpositions 171
        2. Producing abortion.. 172
    II. In labor.. 172
        1. In normal labor... 172
        2. In malpositions... 172
        3. In the expression of the placenta......................... 173
    III. In childbed... 173
E—THE DEVELOPMENT OF EXTERNAL MANIPULATIONS IN RECENT
    OBSTETRIC PRACTICE.. 173
LITERATURE.. 175

CHAPTER V.

CHARACTERISTIC LABOR SCENES AMONG THE YELLOW, BLACK AND RED RACES.

MONGOLIANS.. 177
    Japanese.. 177
    Karafuto Ainos.. 180
        Position.. 181
        Delivery of child.. 182
        Placenta... 182
    Calmucks.. 183
NEGROES.. 185
    Religious ceremonies and superstitions................................. 185
    Pregnancy... 186
    Parturition.. 186
    Afterbirth... 187
    Lactation and childbed... 187
RED RACES.. 189
    Indians of the Pacific Coast... 191
        Preparation.. 191
        Labor, simple and complicated... 191
        After-treatment.. 194
            Walking and compressing abdomen..................................... 194
            Lying near fire warmly wrapped.. 195

PAGE

Eastern Tribes.. 196
   Shelter for confinement.. 197
   Delivery.. 198
   Medical treatment.. 199
   Management of afterbirth... 200
   Five day periods.. 202
   No flesh eaten by husband 202

LIST OF

ILLUSTRATIONS.

FIG.   PAGE

1—Funeral Urn with Ancient Peruvian Labor Scene ....Frontispiece.

2—Labor Scene among the Wakambas (western portion of central
   Africa) 13

3—Mythical Labor Scene from Academy of Medicine in New York 14

4—Brulé-Sioux, standing.. 15

5—Ceram, standing, semi-suspended.. 17

6—Southern Negress, suspended.. 19

7—Sioux Squaw, seated cross-legged on the ground........................ 22

8—Pawnee Labor, squatting, back to back...................................... 24

9—Squatting Posture of the Tonkawas.. 25

10—Obstetric Position of the Persians—From Ploss (after Pollak and
    Hæntsche)... 27

11—Southern Negress, kneeling, arms resting on chair..................... 29

12—Blackfoot Squaw, kneeling, resting upon a staff......................... 32

13—Comanche Labor, with Scene of Surroundings............................ 34

14—Chippewa Labor, kneeling, inclined backwards........................... 37

15—Framework formerly in use in Japan for the support of the partu-
    rient in a kneeling posture... 38

16—Sitting posture of the Japanese, customary in child-bed............. 39

17—Kootenai Squaw, knee-face position with assistant astraddle...... 42

18—Images from the period of the Mound Builders........................... 46

19—Northern Mexico.. 47

20—Coyotero Apaches, difficult Labor... 48

21—Kaffir Woman in Labor.. 52

22—Oronoko Indian, seated semi-recumbent in hammock.................. 54

23—Labor Scene in Ancient Greece, group in the Cesnola Collection,
    New York... 56

24—Modern Cypriote midwife's chair, Cesnola................................. 57

25—The Scientific Posture Advocated in the 16th Century. From Joan-
    nes Michaelis Savonarola, 1547... 59

FIG.   PAGE

26—The Obstetric Couch in the Rural Districts of Ohio in 1845 61

27—Semi-recumbent in the Husband's Lap, assistants holding hands and knees, Virginia 63

29—Andemanese Labor Scene 65

30—Origin of the Obstetric Chair (Engelmann) 66

31—Development of the Obstetric Chair (from Goodell). Chairs of Savonarola, 1547; Eucharius Rhodius, 1544; Deventer, 1701; Stein 1805 67

32—Delivery in the Obstetric Chair; after Ruefflus, 1637 70

33—Obstetric Chair now in use in Syria 72

34—Favorite Posture of the French Canadian 74

35—Japanese Labor. Instrumental Delivery 75

36—Penomonee Labor 76

37—Birth of the Emperor Titus, from Ploss, after an antique painting on the ceiling of a room in the Palace of Titus, on the Esquiline Hill in Rome 77

38—Labor Scene in the Rural Districts of Virginia; semi-recumbent in bed 78

39—Couch and Lying-in Chamber of the Siamese. From Ploss 81

40—Crow Creek. Prone upon face and abdomen, across a pillow 83

41—Semi-recumbent, in the agony of the expulsive effort 86

42—Kneeling, clinging to rope 90

43—Manual Expression of the Placenta. Penomonee Indian 101

44—Use of the Squaw's Belt. Sioux Indian 105

45—Placental Expression as Practiced by the Indians of the Uintah Valley Agency 106

46—Placental Expression: Mexico 108

47—Vessels in which the Placenta is Buried: Japan 113

48—Temporary Shelter for the Lying-in Woman: Comanches 127

49—Japanese Lying-in Couch and Supports used in Child-bed 129

50—Bandage as Used in Mexico 162

51—Management of Difficult Labor in Siam 164

52—Massage and Expression as Practiced in Mexico 167

53—Position of Japanese Woman in Labor and Arrangement of her Couch 179

54—Kiowa Labor, drawn by a Kiowa Indian 190

55—Mexican Indian in Labor, showing posture of patient and assistants. From photograph taken near San Luis Potosi, by Dr. G. Barroeta. 193

56—Kiowa Midwife blowing an emetic into patient's mouth. Drawn by a Kiowa Indian 198

ERRATA.

Menominee.................p. 23, 112, etc., should read...............Menemonee.
Wazahzak.................. ....p. 26, " " ....Wazahzah.
Agallala..... ....26, 100, etc., " " .... Ogallala.
Clatsops.................. .... 31, 99, etc., " " .... Klatsops.
Cataraugus................................ 31, etc., " " ....Catarangus.
Calmucks .... " " .... Kalmucks.
Uncpapas.....................33, 99, 110, etc., " " ....Uncapapas.
Unitah............. ....33, 35, 105, etc., " " ....Uintah, or Uinta.
Childbirth...............39, under Fig. 16, " " ....Childbed.
Fig. 16.............................. ....46, " " ....Fig. 18.
Yanktonans................. ....99 etc.. " " .... Yanktonais.
Umpynas...................................99, " " ....Umpanas.
Kootewais................ ....99, " " ....Kootenais.
Commanches............ . ...99, " " .... Comanches.
Rus ....103, 109, etc., " " ....Rees.

CONTENTS

CHAPTER I.

POSTURE IN LABOR.

INTRODUCTION.—

Origin of this paper—Ancient Peruvian Urn—Rigby—Ploss—Ludwig —How to study the natural position of women in labor—Plan of this investigation—Conclusions reached—Thanks for assistance rendered—Geographical distribution of the various positions.

PART I.

POSITION OF PARTURIENT WOMEN among peoples whose parturition is governed by instinct and not by modern obstetrics—Savages of to-day and civilized races of the past.

PERPENDICULAR OR UPRIGHT POSTURE—Standing—common among Sclavonians and Silesians—in India and parts of Africa—Partially suspended—Suspended.

INCLINED POSITIONS — Sitting erect, rare—Squatting — Indians — Tunis and Persia—Kneeling—quite common, especially yellow and red races—Kneeling with the body inclined forward—Typical description of labor seen among Comanche Indians by Maj. Forwood—Shelter erected—Hot douche—Curious Japanese custom—Knee-elbow positions—In difficult cases in middle ages—Kootenais—Kneeling with the body erect, inclined backwards or partially suspended —Tartars—Supposed to have existed among the mound-builders or pre-historic people of America—Coyotero. Apaches in difficult labor—Cases in which precise description is lacking—"Why did not the knees of my mother remain stiff and I strangle in birth?"—Semi-recumbent — Frequent among ancients — Sitting semi-recumbent —Indians—Kaffirs—Arabs—Ancient group from Cesnola collection—Still practiced in Cyprus—Modern cypriote midwife's chair—Sitting on the lap—Same advocated by Savonarola, 1547—Peculiar couch for same position in Ohio—Virginia—The Obstetric Chair—Origin—History—Development—Described in the "generation and birth of man"—Rocking chair in use in Syria—Semi-recumbent, strictly speaking—Canada—Japan—Penomonee Indians—Ancient Rome.

HORIZONTAL OR RECUMBENT—Ordinary dorsal decubitus—Care among primitive peoples—Lateral decubitus—In isolated cases—Prone upon stomach—Rare—Sometimes in difficult labor.

PART II.

THE POSITION OF WOMEN AMONG CIVILIZED RACES OF THE PRESENT DAY IN THE AGONY OF THE EXPULSIVE PAINS—Semi-recumbent position usually taken.

RESUME AND CONCLUSIONS—Instinct governs position of savages—Comfort and modesty govern modern obstetrics—Positions vary in different stages of labor—Striking positions mostly in last stage—Massage in difficult cases—We should give patients greater liberty in labor—Dorsal decubitus undesirable as a rule—An inclined position should be resorted to—Semi-recumbent best.

CHAPTER II.

THE THIRD STAGE OF LABOR.

TREATMENT OF SIMPLE CASES—More natural among primitive people—Mostly the placenta is delivered in the same position in which the child was expelled—Manual expression—Kneeding of the abdomen very common—Diaphragm often made use of—Traction on the cord not as common as among civilized people—Less often is the placenta delivered in a position different from the one occupied during the expulsion of the child—The motion, or the standing position assumed, supposed to further expulsion.

MANAGEMENT OF DIFFICULT AND COMPLICATED CASES—Forcible expulsion by external pressure—Methods of cutting and tying the cord—Burial of after-birth and other superstitions—Importance of skilled management in the third stage—Vis a Tergo practiced by primitive people—a position only recently obtained by scientific Midwifery.

CHAPTER III.

PREGNANCY, PARTURITION AND CHILDBED.

Many points of resemblance to the customs of a more advanced civilization.

PREGNANCY.—Its importance—Rarity of abortion—Testing the value of conception in the seventh month—Anxiety for male offspring—Signs of pregnancy—Careful treatment of pregnant women—Peculiar superstition of the Pahutes.

LABOR.—Short and easy—Rarity of accidents—Comparison of labor among civilized and savage peoples—The most common accidents—Their treatment—Special rooms or huts used—Superstitions—Labor usually private—Couch used—Old women, occasionally so-called midwives assist the parturient—In difficulties a priest or medicine man is summoned—Assistance is simple—Various external manipulations—Towel about abdomen — Expression — Rubbing — Fright—Teas and herbs.

CHILDBED. — Immediately after delivery some walk about — Others plunge into a lake or river—warm water used by Sclavonians—Fire —A binder rare—Time of rest accorded is brief—Immediate work among some peoples—Diet rarely changed—Some medicines are used—Father sometimes dieted—Free flow of lochia encouraged—Sickness rare — Child dipped into cold water — Strapped on board —Kanikars apply child at once to breast—Kalmucks and others do not suckle for first three to five days—Period of nursing varies from two to five years—Weaning by asafetida—Poor food cause of sickness and death—Kinds of food given the child—Medicines used.

CHAPTER IV.

MASSAGE AND EXPRESSION.

HISTORY OF MASSAGE.—Spoken of in history and poetry—Advocated by Hippocrates—Popular in Sweden—Manipulations numerous and well-defined—Stimulation of muscle and nerve one of its most important physiological effects.

EXTERNAL MANIPULATIONS LONG USED IN OBSTETRIC PRACTICE.—The only means a crude people have of overcoming difficulties in labor—Resorted to in all possible positions—Shampou—Cong-Fou—Ambouk.

EXTERNAL MANIPULATIONS NOW IN USE.—Numerous—1. *Simple compression and expression*—By the arms of an assistant—Kneeling or sitting behind the patient the assistant uses his arms as a compressor—See Frontispiece—A bandage passed around the body is tightened by an assistant—The abdomen is drawn across a rope or pole—The abdomen stripped down by arms of assistants—Expression by means of the feet—Pressure upon a staff—Lying upon the stomach. 2. *Massage*—A more complicated manipulation—The patient shaken upon a blanket, in the air—Permanent pressure—The uses of massage and expression—In pregnancy—To correct malpositions—To produce abortion—In labor—Even in simple cases—To change position of child—To hasten expulsion of placenta—In childbed rare--The development of external manipulations in recent obstetric practice—Wiegand, 1812—Wright—Braxton Hicks—Credé—Literature.

CHAPTER V

CHARACTERISTIC LABOR SCENES AMONG THE YELLOW, BLACK, AND RED RACES.

YELLOW RACES.—*Japanese* use binder during pregnancy—School for midwives—Kneel in labor—Variance of customs when the child is male or female—Value of the remnant of the cord. *Ainos*—roomy pelvis—Preparations for labor—Delivery—Girdle applied after expulsion of child—hemorrhages not rare from pulling out placenta. *Kalmucks*—Squat—Firing of gun to hasten expulsion—Mother unclean for three weeks—Burial of placenta—Nursing up to future pregnancy.

BLACK RACES.—*Loango Negroes* above average—Women considered unclean during menstruation and childbed—Loango women short-breasted—A moral people—" Ndodschi"—Parturition easy—Patient stands, leaning against a wall, or kneels—Prone upon stomach in difficult cases—Gag in mouth and nose to force expulsion—Superstition as to placenta and cord —Frequent bathing—Massage—Sexual intercourse—Love of the Loango mother for her child—Baptism.

THE RED RACES.—Kneeling posture most common. *Indians of the Pacific Coast*—Move about in first stage—Compression of abdomen—Semi-recumbent, but kneeling in difficult cases—Uterus assisted in immediately expelling the placenta—Some walk about after delivery—Compress abdomen—Others are wrapped in blankets—Placed by fire—No puerperal diseases. *Eastern Tribes*—Peculiar shelter constructed by Comanches—Disgusted at examination—Ceremonies aiding labor—Effect of fear—Cord tied one foot from body—Peculiar method of paying the doctor—Superstitions as to woman's functions—Mother and father refrain from meat—Description of last three illustrations.

PREFACE.

———

In offering these pages to the Profession, I must ask their indulgence, as well as a kindly consideration, for a work which is novel in kind; and lest the gentle critic, with a keen pen, should in his friendly way point out to the reader the palpable faults of my little book, I will at once crave his indulgence for presenting a subject *ethnological*—rather than *medical*—in character, and for giving the work to the public with the present faulty arrangement of Chapters.

In the Introduction to Chapter I., I will tell how an examination of that ancient Peruvian Funeral Urn incited me to the study of the customs of Primitive Peoples—at first only of the position occupied by Women in Labor, the subject which would, perhaps, most naturally arouse curiosity and stimulate research on account of the peculiar and very striking facts presented.

So many other strange and interesting, mostly unknown, data accumulated from the responses which my enquiries received from all quarters of the Globe and from the perusal of the many volumes, Medical, Historical and Ethnological, for which I had ransacked the libraries East and West, that one subject after the other presented itself, and in my enthusiasm I developed one after the other. The result was a series of articles upon subjects ethnological, as I have said, rather than medical, which have been gathered in this little book.

Virchow, that leader and master mind, was one of the first, certainly the first of medical men, to develop the science of ethnology, although more with reference to craniology and sociology, yet thus it has become an ally, a

sister science to medicine; why should we not take one
step farther? Why should ethnology not prove an aid in
the development of other branches of medicine as well?
Although a new departure, I may say that Ethnology will
add greatly to the study of obstetric science and its thorough understanding; it will be a guide to the study of
Midwifery, as Comparative Anatomy is to that of Anatomy,
and moreover a necessity to its complete understanding.

I have presented the result of my investigations by reason of their intense interest to me, and because a comparison of the crude methods of Primitive Peoples and Peoples
of former civilizations with the teachings of scientific
obstetrics of to-day are amusing and interesting, but above
all instructive and important. If I have erred, it is my enthusiasm which has carried me away.

So much for the Subject, now for the Arrangement of the
work. The chapters follow, not in logical order, but in
the succession in which chance presented the material, and
the order in which the articles appeared—the first one on
Posture, in the *Transactions of the American Gynecological Society* of 1880; the second, third and fourth in the
American Journal of 'Obstetrics from April, 1881, to July,
1882; and the fifth in the *Courier of Medicine* of St. Louis
for March and May, 1882.

In the arrangement of this volume circumstances necessitated the faulty order, which the reader *cannot overlook*,
yet will, I trust, *generously pardon*.

Let us glance hastily over some of the more striking
features here presented: Is it not a matter of interest to
see how the *moon*, the world over, is connected with the
menstruation of woman; how, in France, in past centuries
our "*monthly* flow," the German "*Monatliche* Reinigung,"
was called the "tribute which woman renders the *moon;*"
the Indian speaks of a woman in this state as having
"*moon* in the ass"—so the world over. Again, the idea of
cleansing, purifying, is expressed in the German "monatliche *Reinigung*," whilst the natives of Africa, of India,
and of our Western territories, still consider the female at

that time as *unclean*, and isolate her, keep her away, especially from men, in a separate hut ; and that she may be well known to all, when she mingles with others, she is obliged to wear certain well-marked colors during the continuance of the period. This is more particularly the case among the numerous, still natural people of Asia, as it was my good fortune to observe myself among the Nauch girls while traveling in this country. This idea of uncleanliness clings equally to the puerpera during the continuance of the lochial flow, and, remarkable enough, in a different degree to the *lochia rubra* and *alba*.

How reasonable ! The menstruating woman is confined in a separate hut, is isolated, does no work, rests, is not exposed to cold or exertion, and thus escapes the numerous uterine troubles which befall the civilized female by reason of ignorant or careless exposure during this period of increased sensitiveness.

The parturient is confined in an isolated shelter, which is destroyed when labor is over, or in a hut or house kept for the purpose, in a particular room. Whatever the idea may be, the result is certainly to prevent infection—to prevent puerperal fever.

The Japanese in pregnancy already endeavor to prevent malpositions by external manipulations of the abdomen; others bind the abdomen in pregnancy. How sensible their laws governing coition during pregnancy ! we can certainly, with advantage, study their reasonable, though instinctive and crude customs !

A vast and important fund of knowledge may be derived from a study of the various positions occupied by women of different peoples in their labors. According to their build, to the shape of the pelvis, they stand, squat, kneel or lie upon the belly ; so also they vary their position in various stages of labor according to the position of the child's head in the pelvis. Does the great number of natural labors resulting not point to a law greatly at variance with the teachings of modern obstetrics ? Is it not evident that different positions should be given in different stages of labor, and in its various periods? But it will necessitate a great advance in obstetric science and much research to determine the underlying law. Here, however, we have the facts.

Although primitive peoples, like modern obstetricians, vary in the method of managing the third stage of labor, manual expression is almost universally resorted to; the *vis a tergo* is acknowledged, and the cord rarely serves the injurious purpose to which most modern midwives put it. As I say at the conclusion of chapter III., the North American Indians and the African Negroes, undoubtedly other tribes also, have for ages followed a practice so perfect that only within the last few years the most alert of our obstetricians are in a position to compare with them. This fact has been noticed by Dr. C. M. Fenn, of San Diego, California, who has an article in the *American Journal of Obstetrics* for 1881 contemptuously termed the "Practice and Perils of Belly-squeezing in Mexican Obstetrics," in which he tells of their rude ways, and at the close is greatly astonished that no harm is done, but that the women do well. He says : " Convalesence has been rapid and normal in all of the cases which have come under my observation, and sufficient time has elapsed (more than six months since the last case) for the development of uterine ailments. More than this, in a not limited experience among these people, I have met with but two or three cases of uterine disease, and am prepared to assert that metritis, oöphoritis, and kindred maladies, are exceptionally rare."

How grand a proof from unwilling source to the eficiency of this method which scientific obstetricians are just beginning to adopt, in fact, have just discovered. Massage and expression, external manipulations, have reached such a perfection as uncultured minds can give : we can learn much from the customs of these people, and if developed by science, sifted and classified, great good will result.

The savage mother, the Negress, the Australian or

Indian, still governed by her instinct, is far in advance of the ordinary woman of our civilization. She bathes herself and her offspring at once, she keeps herself clean. Wonderful to say, the same difference exists among the various races of Primitive People in their customs as to nursing as we find among the physicians of to-day. Some few put the child to the breast at once, most wait for two or three days, and of milk fever they seem to know nothing ; the time of nursing also varies greatly, usually from one to two years. Their methods of weaning are like our own, in the application of asafœtida to the nipple, or of charcoal, to disgust the child ; even the castor-bean plant has been used as a lactagogue, the mother washing her breast with its juice.

I have but briefly referred to some of the interesting points to show how similar the obstetric practices of Primitive Peoples, past and present, are to our own, and yet although crude how far in advance in many points—in all such in which simpler means, the hands and external manipulations will answer. The womb they never enter, instruments they have none, but as far as general treatment and external manipulations will reach their management is wonderful, and we will find much to study, to imitate, and to develop.

The great field opened to us is the study of the position to be occupied by woman in labor, as determined by the configuration of her pelvis and the position of the child's head. Primitive peoples have solved this problem by virtue of their instinct ; now it remains for the science of civilized races to determine the when and wherefore.

I trust that what I have said may induce the reader to peruse these pages with a certain interest which will lead him to pardon or forget their faulty arrangement.

G. J. E.

3003 Locust Street,
St. Louis, June 1, 1882.

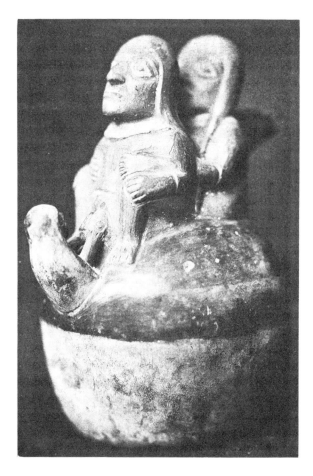

FIG. I.

FUNERAL URN, WITH ANCIENT PERUVIAN LABOR SCENE.

POSTURE IN LABOR.

It was my good fortune in 1877 to add a valuable collection of ancient Peruvian pottery to my archeological museum. At the same time, whilst interested in these matters, I was told of an urn or vessel brought from the ancient graves of Peru, which represented a midwife delivering a woman in labor, and was then stowed away in the home of its discoverer, Dr. Coates, of Chester, Penn. My interest was at once aroused and I wrote to the gentleman requesting a photograph or cast of this unique piece of pottery. I received no answer, but constantly bore the subject in mind, until, finally, upon my visit East in 1879, my esteemed friend, Dr. Albert H. Smith, of Philadelphia, enabled me, through the kind offices of Dr. Anna E. Broomall, to examine the specimen, which proved so intensely interesting to me that I determined to satisfy myself as to the correctness and the historic value of this group, and, moreover, to study the subject of posture in labor. This ancient Peruvian funeral urn, well characterized in the heliotype which accompanies this article, is one of the oldest distinct and well authenticated representations of a labor case which is extant. The method of delivery followed by those, at that time, highly civilized people, a thousand or more years ago, seemed to me so peculiar that I was anxious to know whether other people had similar curious customs and whether any traces of these could be found at the present day; moreover, it appeared to me as if a study of obstetric customs among the more primitive people might lead to valuable results which would serve to guide the practice of the present day. My interest was thoroughly aroused, and by the kind offices of the gentlemen in charge of the Library in the Surgeon-general's office its fund of well-arranged material was kindly placed at my disposal, so that I was enabled at once to enter upon the study of the subject which had so deeply engrossed my attention. I found an extensive literature relating to the subject of posture in labor, but it turns entirely upon the discussion of the relative merits of the dorsal decubitus, as practised upon the continent of Europe and in America, and the left lateral position, which is favored in England ; perhaps, also, the knee-elbow position may come into question, but the discussions are entirely confined to the merits of those positions which are taught by modern obstetric law, and enforced in all civilized communities of the present day where scientific medicine rules. Some had gone beyond this and had attempted to determine the natural position of woman in labor by the study of the position which had been occupied by unfortunate girls, in concealed or secret parturition ; thus Schütz,[1] and Dr. Cohen v. Bæren in Posen, who cites one hundred such cases ; fifty of which occurred in unusual positions : thirty standing, eighteen crouching or squatting, and two kneeling. Of the fifty cases recorded by Schütz, thirty-two — over half — occupied abnormal positions : fourteen standing, sixteen crouching or squatting, two kneeling. Nægele, on the contrary, sought to discover the natural position in labor by secretly observing the movements of an inexperienced girl who was left alone, while in pains, in a room furnished with a bed, chair, sofa, and an obstetric chair. The girl took all possible positions and was finally delivered tossing about on the bed ; she had sought the obstetric chair but gave it up after a moment's trial which appeared so conclusive to her mind that she did not repeat the attempt. Hohl [2] in his clinic made an attempt to see whether women could be confined standing, and, though a great many had been urged to try,

---

[1] *Verhandl. d. Gesellsch. f. Geburtsh. in Berl.*, iv., page 37.
[2] *Lehrb. d. Geburtsh.*, 2 Aufl., Leipzig, 1862, page 114.

only one, induced by a considerable bribe, had been able to complete her labor in this position ; hence, he concluded that all accounts of women being thus confined must be false — an erroneous conclusion, as I shall hereafter show. The first who departed from the beaten track and entered upon the proper course to determine the natural position of women in labor, namely, by historical and ethnological researches, was Rigby, in his paper, published in the " Medical Times and Gazette," for 1857,[1] " What is the natural Position of Women During Labor ? " He refers to the methods previously followed, then traces those peculiar positions which are still customary in secluded parts of England, Scotland, Wales, and Ireland, and seems to come to the conclusion that accidental circumstances determine in a great measure the position which the unassisted woman assumes when seized with violent pains effecting the expulsion of the child ; that she probably walks or tosses about, finally to be delivered in a recumbent position ; and rather seems to indorse the views of his West India correspondent, " That there is no natural position, in labor, for the native women, any more than for a man with colic or a West India dry belly."

The next and most complete work on the subject was by Dr. H. H. Ploss,[2] " Ueber die Lage und Stellung der Frau wæhrend der Geburt bei verschiedenen Völkern." He, without entering upon a theoretical discussion of the question, gives us the results of his very thorough study of the positions occupied by women in labor among the ancients and among the uncultured and savage races of the present day. He recognizes the positions assumed as : *Firstly*, recumbent in a more or less horizontal position. *Secondly*, sitting : (*a*.) in bed ; (*b*.) on a stool ; (*c*.) on a chair ; (*d*.) on a cushion ; (*e*.) on the thighs of another individual. *Thirdly*, standing. *Fourthly*, kneeling. *Fifthly*, squatting. *Sixthly*, swinging. *Seventhly*, suspended in an erect posture. I shall not infrequently refer to the authorities quoted by Dr.

[1] Vol. xv., page 345.
[2] Leipzig, 1872.

Ploss, although in some cases the details of reports, which I have obtained, vary decidedly from the often very meagre statements made by him; and in other cases he has based his assertions upon very questionable and indefinite accounts of travelers, which he has evidently made use of in order to make his paper as complete as possible. In the main it is a sound paper showing a great deal of profound research among the best of authorities, ancient and modern. ‑ I cannot, however, agree with his conclusion, namely, "that among the majority of people ·the parturient women assume the recumbent position." He seems to think that, though not necessarily in an entirely horizontal position, she is delivered lying upon a bed or a couch of some kind.

I might add that in 1870, a paper appeared in Breslau, by H. v. Ludwig,[1] in which the author, upon theoretical grounds, advocates the kneeling or squatting positions to be assumed during the expulsion of the child, and insists that the women of savage races, of people who still exist under the most natural conditions, instinctively assume these positions. As soon as my attention had been once directed to this subject by that remarkable funeral urn, representing the custom of the ancient Peruvians, and I had entered upon the study of the posture occupied during labor by the women of other people, I found a great variety in their customs ; but it soon became evident, and impressed itself forcibly upon my mind, that the *recumbent* position in labor is rarely assumed among those people who live naturally and are, as yet, governed by their instincts and have escaped the influence of civilization and of modern obstetrics. It certainly appeared as if the ordinary obstetric position of to-day must be an unnatural one, and in order to study the question as to what is the natural position of women in labor, the proper and only course to be followed seemed to me to investigate : —

1. The position occupied by women in labor among the

---

[1] " Warum lässt man die Frauen in der Rückenlage gebären ? "

nations of the past; especially among those who boasted of higher civilization.

2. To observe the position assumed by women in labor among savage races of the present day whose movements are still governed by instinct.

I deem it a great mistake that we in this age of culture, should follow custom or fashion so completely, to the exclusion of reason and instinct, in a mechanical act which so nearly concerns our animal nature as the delivery of the pregnant female. If we wish to obtain an idea of the natural position we must look to the woman who is governed by instinct, not by prudery ; and it is only among the savage races that we shall find her at the present day. In this purely animal function instinct will guide the woman more correctly than the varying customs of the times.

3. In our obstetric practice of to-day to observe the movements of women and the positions which ˙they involuntarily assume in the agony of the expulsive pains when instinct comes forward, to the exclusion of every other feeling. I have accordingly—

1. Sought such information as history could give me — as could be afforded by our larger libraries, especially that of the Surgeon-general's office in Washington ; and I have made free use of the references given by Ploss in his work already referred to, and by Goodell,[1] in his instructive paper on " Some Ancient Methods of Delivery."

2. In order to obtain information as to the positions assumed by those people among whom no modern obstetric law or custom as yet prevails — among the savages of the present day — I have corresponded with leading obstetricians in foreign countries, as well as travelers who were likely to assist me in this inquiry. I have sought information from physicians in various portions of our own country, partly by correspondence, partly by questions kindly put to their readers, by a number of our medical journals. The most valuable information, however, I have obtained through circulars sent to the medical officers of the army and the

[1] *Am. J. Obst.*, February, 1872.

physicians to the Indian Agencies, through the Bureau of Ethnology of the Smithsonian Institution in Washington.

3. I have made it my duty to observe the positions assumed by women at the very moment of the expulsion, during the agony of the last pains.

The subject will be divided as follows : —

THE INTRODUCTION.

PART I., treating of the position of women among people whose labor is governed by instinct and not by prudery or the laws of obstetrics.

PART II. The position of women among civilized races of the present day, in the agony of the expulsive pains.

CONCLUSIONS ; and these, I will briefly state, are : that the semi-recumbent and inclined positions are the correct ones for the parturient woman, — anatomically, theoretically, and practically, — and that we have unquestionable ethnological proof of this assertion. We must resume the semi-recumbent position, and it becomes a question whether we should return to the obstetric chair or not.

I have classified the positions, according to the inclination of the axis of the body, into : The perpendicular or upright, the inclined, and the horizontal or recumbent.

A. Perpendicular : —

1. Standing.

2. Partially suspended.

3. Suspended.

B. Inclined : —

1. Sitting erect on stool, cushion, or stone.

2. Squatting, as in defecation.

3. Kneeling.

(*a.*) With the body inclined forward, and resting on a chair or staff.

(*b.*) Knee-elbow position, knee-breast, or knees and hands.

(*c.*) With the body erect or inclined backwards.

(*d.*) Not definitely described.

4. Semi-recumbent.

(*a.*) Sitting semi-recumbent on the ground, a stone, or stool.

(*b.*) On the lap or between the thighs of an assistant who is seated on a chair or on the floor.

(*c.*) The obstetric chair.

(*d.*) Semi-recumbent positions, strictly speaking.

C. Horizontal or recumbent.

(*a.*) On the back.

(*b.*) On the side.

(*c.*) On the chest and stomach.

I have been aided in this work by so many kind friends and fellow practitioners that I feel it my duty to express my thanks to, at least, some of them, for the valuable assistance rendered. Dr. Isaac Coates, formerly of Chester, Penn., gave the impulse to this undertaking by kindly permitting me to photograph the historic urn which he unearthed from its resting place, that it might reveal to us the life of a people long since passed away ; and it is owing to the efforts of Dr. Anna E. Broomall that I was actually enabled to do this. The kindness of Drs. Billings and Fletcher readily enabled me to obtain much important information from the vast and well catalogued materials of the Surgeon-general's library. To Dr. H. C. Yarrow my especial thanks are due for his unceasing efforts in the interest of this undertaking; his position and his researches in the library of the Surgeon-general's office enabled him to extend to me many favors ; with the consent and at the direction of Major J. W. Powell, in charge of the Bureau of Ethnology of the Smithsonian Institution, aided by other friends, he has sent out a series of circulars to the surgeons of the army and Indian Agencies requesting information as to the obstetric practices among our North American Indians; I also gratefully acknowledge my indebtedness to the medical officers of the United States army, and the physicians to the Indian Agencies, for the valuable information given, and their cheerful and generous response to the circular sent. Dr. Raoul Fauquez, of Paris, had the kindness to offer information upon the subject in the various departments of France. Several of our medical journals placed before their readers my questions as to the obstetric practices in remote regions of this country, and numerous professional friends throughout the entire land have given me valuable information as to the country practice in earlier days. Mr. Ad. Bandelier, that ardent archeologist from our neighbor State, gave me an insight into the customs of the natives at the time of the conquest by reference to his valuable library of ancient Spanish authorities. To my friend Dr. C. W. Cooper I owe thanks for valuable assistance rendered throughout the entire work.

Quite a number of the instructive illustrations I owe to the genius of St. Louis' talented artist, Mr. Carl Gutherz; whilst Dr. H. H. Ploss, of Leipzig, has permitted the use of several of the cuts from his own work.

GEOGRAPHICAL DISTRIBUTION.

Europe.

The dorsal decubitus, with the woman recumbent in bed, is now almost universal, having superseded the obstetric chair of the beginning of this century. Peculiar positions are still found here and there in remote districts.

France. A standing position is occasionally assumed.

Italy. Semi-recumbent on the lap ; and in earlier days knee-elbow, semi-recumbent in bed, and erect, clinging to the neck of an assistant.

Spain. Kneeling.

Germany. Standing ; on the lap of an assistant ; partly suspended ; semi-recumbent in bed, or in a sling.

Russia. Erect, wholly suspended ; squatting ; kneeling ; sitting erect and in the lap of an assistant.

Sweden. Recumbent.

Greece. Kneeling and semi-recumbent in bed, or on a low stool reclining against an assistant, in ancient Greece. In later times, recumbent in bed, or semi-recumbent on a low stool, reclining against an assistant, which appears still very common.

Turkey. Chair ; sitting on a stool.

Great Britain. Clinging to the neck of an assistant ; kneeling, arms resting on a chair or in the lap of an assistant ; knee-elbow position ; sitting on a low stool ; squatting ; sitting semi-recumbent in the lap of an assistant (several of these positions have been frequently observed in Irish or Welsh emigrants in this country).

Asia.

Kamtschatka. Kneeling.
Mongolia.` Kneeling.
China. Chair or bed.
Japan. Chair, semi-recumbent, or kneeling erect on the floor.
Philippine Islands. Standing.
Sumatra. Recumbent.
Siam. Recumbent ; lying on the side or back.
Burmah. Recumbent, on the back.
India. Standing; on the lap; sitting on a cushion or stool ; recumbent in bed.
Andaman Islands. In the lap of the husband.
Persia. Squatting or kneeling.
Arabia. Squatting ; semi-recumbent on the chair or the lap ; or on two flat stones clinging to a rope.
Palestine. Chair.
Syria. Rocking-chair ; semi-recumbent.
Hebrews. Semi-recumbent (on stones or a stool) and squatting.
Cyprus. Semi-recumbent on a stool (ancient and modern).

Africa.

Egypt, ancient. Squatting.
Egypt, modern. Chair.
Abyssinia. Kneeling ; sitting on a stone, reclining against an assistant or a tree.
Ethiopia. Kneeling; standing.
Dar-Fur. Standing.
East Africa. Standing ; sitting or squatting.
Somali. Standing, holding on to a rope.
Wakamba. Standing, bent over backwards.
Kaffraria. Squatting.
Hottentots, Cape of Good Hope. Standing.
Old Calabar. Sitting on a chair or block.
Wazegua. Squatting.
Canary Islands. Sitting erect.

North America.

Canada, French settlers. Semi-recumbent on the floor, back against an inclined chair.
Canada, Iroquois. Standing, clinging to the neck.
Mexico, Indians, half-breeds, and lower class of whites. Kneeling, clinging to a rope or the neck ; squatting ; standing, and semi-recumbent on the lap and in bed.
United States, Caucasians descended from various European races. Kneeling ; squatting ; sitting on the husband's lap ; semi-recum-

bent in bed or on the floor, against an inclined chair ; standing, and knee-elbow position.

United States, Negroes.   Kneeling, head in the lap; squatting : suspended from the limb of a tree.

United States, Indians.   Mostly kneeling, clinging to a tent-pole, the body inclined forward, or to a rope or horizontal staff, the body inclined back ; often squatting ; occasionally sitting semi-recumbent in the lap or on the floor ; semi-recumbent, or kneeling erect ; more rarely recumbent ; standing erect, clinging to the neck of an assistant ; tied to a tree, or suspended ; and the knee-chest position.

Central and South America.

Nicaragua.   Kneeling.
Guatemala.   Squatting.
Venezuela.   Semi-recumbent, seated in a hammock.
Peru, ancient and modern.   Semi-recumbent in the husband's lap.
Chili.   Semi-recumbent in the lap.
Brazil.   Recumbent on the ground or in a hammock.

Australia and Surrounding Islands.

Australia.   Sitting erect ; recumbent.
Ceram.   Standing erect ; suspended.
Polynesia.   Squatting.
West Micronesia.   Squatting.
New Zealand.   Kneeling.
Sandwich Islands.   Semi-recumbent on the lap, or lying on a mat.

PART I.

Position of Parturient Women among People whose Parturition is governed by Instinct and not by Modern Obstetric Fashion. — Among the Ancients. — Among the Savage or Uncivilized Races of the present Day, and in Remote Districts of Civilized Countries.

I HAVE, as already stated, determined to classify the various positions, as nearly as possible, in accordance with the position assumed by the axis of the body, and shall hence consider first: A. The Perpendicular or Upright Positions; then B. The Inclined Positions; and finally C. The Horizontal or Recumbent Positions.

A. PERPENDICULAR OR UPRIGHT POSTURE.

Under this heading I shall discuss, individually, those positions in which the body is erect or almost so, and, in accordance with some slight variations, will distinguish: 1. *The Standing*, 2. *The Partially Suspended*, 3. *The Entirely Suspended Positions.*

1. STANDING.

We shall find this apparently uncomfortable position assumed even at the present day, and in our own country: Thus, Dr. H. F. Campbell, of Georgia, writes me that he has delivered a patient standing, clinging to the bed-post, who would rather dispense with his services than assume any other position. Among our Indians it is rarely observed, although I have been informed by a correspondent that the Sioux women are delivered standing erect; I think that we shall find a partially erect, partially standing, position more frequent among them. The natives of the Antilles, if we may accept so venerable an authority as Fray Juan de Torquemada, are confined standing, but also at times assume the kneeling or recumbent postures. In France it seems to have been quite a common position in some of the interior departments, as Godefroy [1] warns his colleagues never to permit the women to be confined in a standing posture, as hemorrhage, prolapse of the uterus, and rupture of the perineum are more apt to ensue than in any other. During the past century it seems to have been the most common position among the Sclavonians in the mountainous regions of upper Silesia, where, in 1747, a physician, in his book on midwifery, even advises such patients as do not wish to be confined in bed to assume this position, with some strong person supporting them from behind and holding their arms, whilst others hold the separated legs, and the midwife sits comfortably in front.[2]

The Hindoos, especially upon the eastern coast of India and in the vicinity of Madras, are delivered in an erect, standing posture, supported by an assistant under each shoulder — the midwife attending to her duties, being seated in front of the patient,[3] and whether rare or not at the present day the position is certainly traditionary, as bas-reliefs still exist upon the ancient Indian monuments which represent the act of delivery in this very same way.

In Central Africa, and near the Cape, among the Boers, the standing posture is not uncommon. Among the Negritos, upon the Philippine Islands, the parturient woman assumes the standing position, but apparently bent forward a little, as she supports the abdomen against a bamboo cane planted in the ground, thus apparently exercising some pressure upon the uterus.[4]   Among the Wakambas, in Africa,

---

[1] *Revue de thérap. méd.-chir.*, Par., 1864, No 9, page 227.   Ploss, p. 38.

[2] Ploss, *Die Lage und Stellung der Frau während der Geburt*, Leipzig, 1872, p. 38.

[3] J. A. Roberton, *opprak. jutschr.*, 1847, v. 6.   H. B. French.

[4] Mallat, *Les Philippines*, 1846.   *Ztschr. f. Ethn.*

the patient assumes the standing posture assisted by two friends, but bends over backwards, and a third is seated in front to receive the child.[1]

A similar position is shown in an old painting in the Academy of Medicine in New York. (See Fig. 3.) The

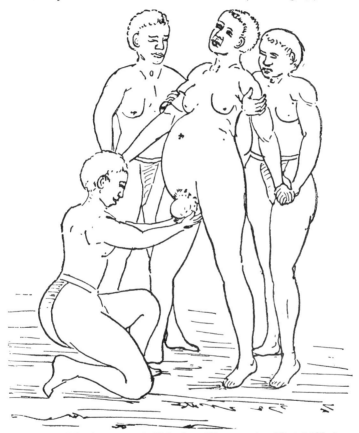

FIG. 2. — Labor Scene among the **Wakambas.** (Western portion of Central Africa.)

history of this picture, which represents some mythical or mythological scene, I cannot trace, but the artist has certainly depicted the custom of his period in the position

[1] J. M. Hildebrandt, " Ethnographische Notizen über Wakamba und ihre Nachbaren," *Ztschr. f. Ethn.*, Berl., 1878, vol. x., page 394.

assumed by the parturient. For this reason it has appeared to me of sufficient interest to place it side by side with the labor scene among the less fanciful Wakambas.

The Loangos, in Equatorial Africa, are delivered standing, leaning against the wall of the hut, or kneeling, the head resting upon the arms. The reason assigned for this procedure is that they expect to obtain the desired head presentation by assuming these positions. In difficult labor

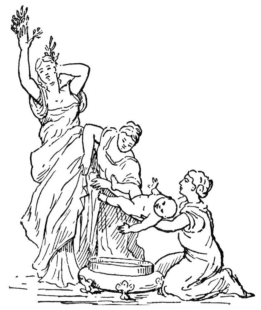

FIG. 3. — Mythical Labor Scene.

the patient is placed upon her face and chest, and finally upon her back, and choked and kneaded until an expulsion in some direction is accomplished.[1]

2. PARTIALLY SUSPENDED.

Parturient women endeavor to assume this position of partial suspension in various ways. Some hang to the neck

[1] *Indiscretes aus Loango.* Dr. Peschuel-Loesche. *Ztschr. f. Ethn.*, 1878, x., p. 29.

of a husband or friend, others swing themselves by a rope from the branch of a tree, while some are tied up until the act is over, as if undergoing punishment. The squaws of the Brulé Sioux, the largest branch of the great Sioux Nation, are confined in the midst of a crowd of indifferently solicitous relatives and friends, one or more matrons always being present as midwives. In the first stage of labor, that is, prior to the expulsion of the *liquor amnii*, the squaw sits or lies upon the ground groaning vociferously ; during the expulsion of the fetus, her posture is erect or nearly so, with her arms about the neck of a stout male supporter, and I am informed upon credible authority that the young bachelor bucks are most frequently chosen for this service.

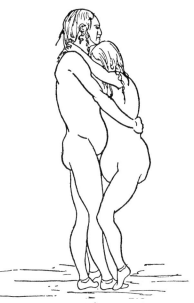

FIG. 4. — Brulé Sioux. Standing.

The women of the Iroquois in Canada, are all confined standing, generally leaning on a friend's shoulder, whilst the child is taken by the midwife behind the patient. The position is probably the same as described among the Sioux.

In Japan this position is resorted to in the attempt to correct malpositions in the earlier months of pregnancy. The Japanese medical man makes the patient stand up and put her arms around his neck ; he then presses his shoulder against her breast, and his knees between hers in such a manner that she is firmly supported, and, while in this position he manipulates, performing lateral massage with his hands, beginning with the seventh cervical vertebra and bringing them downward and forward, snapping his fingers to distract the attention of the woman. Finally, he rubs the natés and hips with the palms of the hands forwards, beginning at the sacrum, and repeating the movement sixty or seventy times. This process is repeated every morning after the fifth month.[1]

The " New York Medical Record" adds, that the accoucheurs are, in Japan, as a rule, advanced in age. If this custom is found in our own country it certainly comes to us from some of the inland countries of Europe. Thus, Spence, in his " System of Midwifery,"[2] says that the position which is very frequently practised in the northern portion of Scotland, is that of hanging about the neck of a person as tall, or, if possible, taller than herself, who gently supports the patient's back, and with her knees fixes the knees of the woman in labor. In Italy it was Savonarola, who died in Padua in 1460, who taught that in difficult labors the parturient woman should either hang to the neck of a stout person or assume the knee-elbow position.[3]

The practice in some Mexican families [4] is to keep the woman in an upright position, with the knees and thighs slightly flexed, the feet wide apart, while she supports herself by two ropes suspended from above. He adds that massage is very freely resorted to, but no binder is at any time used.

We find precisely the same position in Africa among several native tribes. Thus, the Somali women assume an erect posture, partially suspended by a rope during the expulsion of the child, which is received by a family attendant or midwife.[5] So, also, we find that the women of Dar Fur, on the Nile, are delivered standing, with the legs separated,[6] holding on to a rope.

---

[1] *La France médicale.*
[2] Edinburgh, 1784.
[3] Siebold, vol. i., page 352.   Ploss, page 44.
[4] Dr. Joseph K. Carson, post-surgeon at Fort Yuma, Cal.
[5] J. M. Hildebrandt, *Ztschr. f. Ethn.*, 1878, vol. x.
[6] " Dar Fur on Nile," *Skizze der Nil Länder,* 1866, page 405.

A somewhat more barbarous custom is that followed by some of our North American Indians, and by the inhabitants of Ceram, an island north of Australia, namely : they tie the patient to a post or tree, with the hands above the head. The Coyoteros are in the habit of tying their women, in labor, to a tree, with the hands above the head,

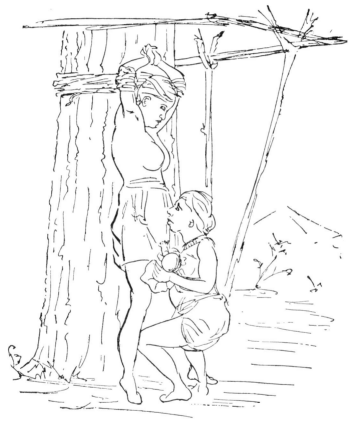

FIG. 5. Ceram. Standing, semi-suspended.

and leave them in this position until the child is born. This cruelty does not appear to affect them in any perceptible manner, and they recover from it in a much shorter time, and resume their avocations sooner, than the most ro-

2

bust white women.[1] The natives of Ceram hastily construct
a rude hut of leaves and brush for the parturient woman,
and an old hag, who assists as midwife, ties the patient,
with her arms as high as possible, to a tree, so that the
balls of the feet barely touch the ground, whilst she herself
takes a more comfortable position before the parturient,
and receives the child in a large leaf, a mat, or an old piece
of cloth. Labor over, the young mother washes herself, or
takes a bath, and immediately returns to her village and to
work.[2]

3. SUSPENDED.

Not unfrequently the negroes in our southern States
still follow the customs brought from their African homes,
or merely handed down by tradition ; in their method of
delivery they do not vary from that of the tribe from which
they sprang. Occasionally the erect posture is taken, and
a graphic description of such a labor has been given me,
as witnessed in Louisiana. A negress gave birth to a
child while hanging on to the limb of a tree. She would
raise herself from the ground during the pains, whilst the
assistant who was with her took charge of the child after it
was born.[3]

In some portions of Finland, among the Esthen, as well
as in some portions of Russia, the women are delivered in
a similar manner while hanging to a cross-bar ; they attempt, as it were, to shake out the child.[4]

We have the authority of *Father Och* that, in Brazil, the
parturient woman occasionally has her arms tied to a tree,
while she is waited on by some old hags until the delivery
is completed.[5]

In some portions of Germany, though the instances are

[1] Dr. W. J. Hoffmann, *Miscellaneous Ethnological Observations
among the Indians in Nevada, Colorado, and Arizona*, p. 471. Hay-
dens' *Survey*, 1876.

[2] Captain Schulze, " Ueber Ceram," *Ztschr. f. Ethn.*, 1877, p. 120.

[3] Dr. A. V. Forquey, of St. Louis.

[4] Kredel. Ploss, p. 43.

[5] Marr, *Nachr. v. Span. Amerika*, i., 202.

rare, the woman is delivered suspended in the arms of her husband, who seizes her from behind and raises her up, so that she is bent backward to such a degree that the tips of the toes barely touch the ground.[1]

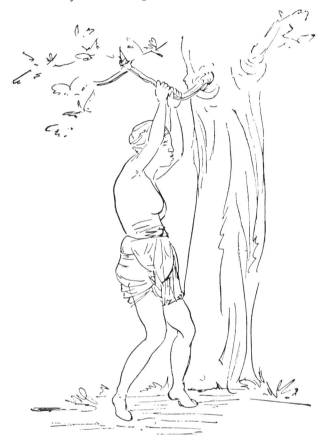

Fig. 6. Southern Negroes. Suspended.

The Siamese, who use massage freely, are usually delivered in the dorsal decubitus ; but in difficult cases, when even tramping upon the abdomen is not attended with success, as a *dernier ressort*, they suspend the patient by means

[1] Hohl, *Midwifery*, second edition, 1862, p. 444.

of a band beneath the arms, and one, sometimes two, of the attendants then clasp with their arms the body of the parturient, and suspend themselves also ; this expedient seldom fails to produce a rupture in some direction, be it the uterus, the perineum, or the encephalon of the child.

B. INCLINED POSITIONS.

This class, which we shall find, by far, the most common among civilized and savage people, ancient and modern, I have divided into four kinds, though the first one may not, perhaps, with the greatest propriety, be called an inclined position.

1. The erect, sitting posture.

2. The squatting position, as in defecation.

3. The kneeling posture and its modifications; and finally, —

4. The semi-recumbent position, whether on the lap of an assistant, in a chair, on the floor, or in bed.

1. SITTING ERECT.

I hardly know whether to consider the erect sitting posture as an inclined or an upright position, but, as the pelvic axis is certainly more inclined than in the standing posture, and, as it will be very hard to draw a line between the distinctly erect sitting posture and the somewhat inclined, I have determined to place it among the inclined, and to consider it first under this head, because it is most nearly related to the perpendicular or upright. Women confined in this position make use of cushions, stones, stools, or mother earth herself ; but the temptation to assume a somewhat reclining position, leaning against the assistant or some other support, is so great, that it is difficult to say with precision that the erect sitting posture is assumed, as the notes upon the subject, by most writers, are not sufficiently clear. I can find but one distinct description of a labor in which it is stated that the patient was confined sitting upright, and that this is the usual position among native

Australians, the weak women only lying down when in labor.[1]

The Nayer women, of Malabar, are confined while seated upon a cushion, or a low three-legged stool without a back, and are supported by the midwife, or some female relative. As is so common among savage races, they then bathe in the nearest stream, or other convenient water, immediately after delivery, and resume their work, as far as is permissible, in the state of uncleanliness in which they are considered to be after labor.[2]

In a similar way the native woman of Guatemala, South America, is confined. She is seated on the ground, supported by a midwife, who presses one knee into the small of her back.[3]

In Calabar, Africa, the same position is assumed, the woman sitting on a low chair, or block, while the midwife squats in front of her, pressing the sides of the abdomen.[4]

On the Canary Islands, the parturient woman sits upon the floor, with a chair or other support beside her, upon which her arms rest. In Astrakhan, in Russia, she sits in a similar way between two boxes or trunks, upon which her arms rest.[5]

A sitting position, with the body decidedly bent forward, was observed in a Sioux squaw, who, like her sisters among most of the Indian tribes, sought a solitary confinement upon the banks of a stream.[6] The position of this woman, until the expulsion of the child, — about forty minutes, — was cross-legged on the floor, her arms crossed over her breast, head bowed, and the body bent forward, especially

---

[1] Hooker, *Journal of the London Ethnological Society*, April, 1869, p. 68.

[2] Herr N. von Miklucko-Macklay, "Anthropologishe Notizen gesammelt auf einer Reise in West Mikronesien und . Nord Milanesien," *Ztschr. f. Ethn.*, 1876, p. 126.

[3] Bernouilli, *Schweiz. Ztschr. f. Heilk.*, Bern, 1864, i. and ii., p. 100. Ploss, *Die Lage und Stellung der Frau während der Geburt*, Leipzig, 1872, p. 20.

[4] Hewan, *Edinb. M. J.*, September, 1864, p. 223.

[5] H. Meyerson. Ploss, p. 20.

[6] Surgeon B. B. Taylor, U. S. A.

during the pains ; the legs were crossed below the knee, and in such a manner that the thighs were widely separated. I may, perhaps, add, though it is of little practical interest, that according to the Egyptologist, Professor Ebers, a

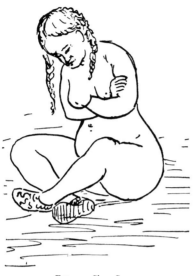

hieroglyph is frequently found on some of the old Egyptian monuments which represents a woman sitting cross-legged, and seems to represent the act of expulsion.[1]

2. SQUATTING.

This position naturally follows the erect sitting posture, although t h e body is always inclined forward to a certain degree ; it is hardly to be defined with exactness, yet we may, in a general way, consider all postures as squatting which

FIG. 7. — Sioux Squaw.

resemble that assumed in defecation. Though apparently inconvenient, and repugnant to the refined woman, this position is certainly the most natural one for expulsion from the abdominal or pelvic viscera, and will certainly, in many cases, facilitate labor. Thus a friend relates his experience : A colored woman, a house servant, carefully reared, who had undergone several very difficult labors, in her fourth or fifth pregnancy, feeling a little uncomfortable, and desiring to be ready, took a pail and went to a pump for water. She carried it for twenty or thirty steps, and, arriving at the gate, felt violent contraction. She set the pail down, squatted, and was delivered of her child.

"So easily she yields her bosom's load,
    You 'd almost think she found it in the road." [2]

[1] Ploss, p. 36.   [2] Dr. Campbell, of Augusta, Ga.

In other confinements she had assumed the squatting position, and was easily delivered.

Then, again, he tells me of attending a lady of good position in society in two labors. "In her first labor, delivery was retarded without apparent cause. There was nothing like impaction, or inertia, yet the head did not advance. At every pain she made violent efforts, and would bring her chest forward. I had determined to use the forceps, but just then, in one of the violent pains, she raised herself up in bed and assumed a squatting position, when the most magic effect was produced. It seemed to aid in completing delivery in the most remarkable manner, as the head advanced rapidly, and she soon expelled the child by what appeared to be one prolonged attack of pain. In subsequent parturition, labor appeared extremely painful and retarded in the same manner; I allowed her to take the same position, as I had remembered her former labor, and she was delivered at once, squatting."

The Irish, also, are familiar with this most natural of all positions, although the knee-elbow position is more common among them. A striking instance is related to me of a poor Irish woman who was found upon a vacant lot in New York city, squatting upon the ground, endeavoring to express the placenta, the child having already been delivered in the same position.[1]

Dr. John Williams, physician to the Green Bay Indian Agency, seems to consider with great favor this position as assumed by the Pawnee Indians. He has had extensive experience as Agency physician, having been associated with different tribes of Indians in different localities, and he does not think that climate has anything to do with the labor of the parturient woman. He says: "I am satisfied that the Pawnee Indian women are far more exempt from the maladies resulting from parturition than the Menomonee, Stockbridge, or Oneidas of Wisconsin. Possibly this may be attributed to the position assumed during labor. The position of the Pawnee woman in parturition is gener-

[1] Dr. F. A. Castle. New York.

ally a squatting one with the Indian woman who assists her squatting at her back, the two being back to back, and the accoucheur, who is generally a medicine man, in front of her upon his knees, with a gourd in one hand, which he rattles constantly, and a pipe in his mouth which he smokes, blowing the smoke under the clothes or covering of the patient until after the delivery of the child." Evidently, a warm vapor bath to soften the parts. Precisely the same position is assumed in West Micronesia, where the mother, during the expulsive pains, assumes a squatting — half-sit-

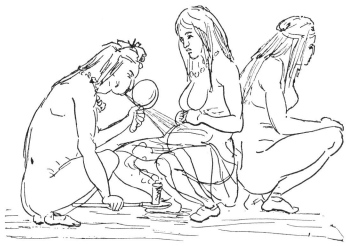

FIG. 8. — Pawnee Labor.

ting, half-lying position, her back resting against the back of an assistant.[1]   So also the Wazequa women squat during labor.[2]

Others of our Indians, than those already mentioned assume this position, with slight variations. Thus [3] the Nez-Percés and Gros-Ventres : during the first stages of

[1] Herr von Micklucko-Macklay, *Ztschr. f. Ethn.*, 1876, page 105, " Anthropologische Notizen," etc.

[2] J. M. Hildebrandt, " Ethnographische Notizen." *Ztschr. f. Ethn.*, 1878, vol. x., page 394.

[3] Major Chas. R. Greenleaf, Surgeon U. S. A.

labor the woman is in a stooping posture, with the buttocks resting on the heels. An assistant places herself back of the patient, clasping her body with her arms, letting the fingers reach below the ribs over the base of the uterus, making steady pressure backwards and outwards during the pains. During the third stage, or expulsion of the child, the patient, however, lies down indifferently on either

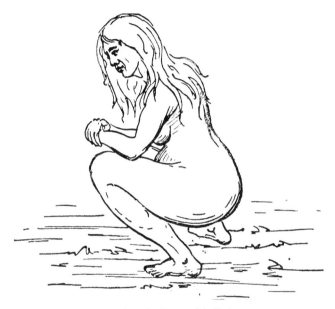

Fig. 9.— Squatting Posture of the Tonkawas.

side or on the back, while the pressure by the hands of the assistant is kept up continuously, if on the side; if on the back, the assistant remains by the side of the patient and keeps up the pressure in the before-mentioned directions. In difficult labors the knee-elbow position is assumed. The Tonkawas retain the squatting posture until after the expulsion of the child:[1] so also the Coyotero or White Mountain Apaches: "The Coyotero squaw occupies any position she pleases, generally standing or walking, until bearing

[1] Wm. R. Steinmetz, Surgeon U. S. A.

down pains supervene, when she assumes the squatting
posture until after the birth of the child and placenta ; but
in tedious cases the patient is suspended in a half-kneeling
position by a lariat from the limb of a tree and the child
stripped out, as it were." [1]

A slight variation of this position is found among some
of the larger branches of the Sioux Nation, the Brulé,
Loafer, Agallala, Wazahzak, and Northern, who stoop, and
with their hands grasp deer-thongs attached to stakes driven
into the ground, against which they pull. [2]

The Mexican half-breeds, in New Mexico and vicinity,
sometimes suspend a cord from the ceiling, with a stick attached, so that the women can seize it in a half-upright,
squatting position. [3]   The same we find among the Kalmucks upon the borders of China and Russia, and not unfrequently during the third stage of labor they squat lower
in bed on their heels, whilst holding with their hands on to
a pole, the abdomen being pressed from behind by an assistant. [4]

The squatting position, with the body bent forward, is
assumed by the women of Southern Arabia in the vicinity
of Aden, who, however, rest their hands upon the ground
instead of crossing them upon the breast, as the squaw
does.   But, among these people, as among so many of our
Indians, and the tribes of Africa, massage is freely resorted
to if any obstruction seems to prevent the labor, sometimes
with the hands, sometimes with the feet ; in the latter case,
the assistant, standing with her heels upon the lower ribs,
works the fundus of the uterus with her toes. [5]

Every people varies its customs a little.   The Polynesian
and Australian negresses squat, as in defecation, over a
small hole which they have scratched in the ground for the
reception of the child. [6]   Ploss also states, upon the author-

---

[1] Walter Reed, M. D., Asst. Surgeon, U. S. A.
[2] W. H. Faulkner, M. D.   [3] H. R. Tilton, Surgeon U. S. A.
[4] Krebel, *Volks Med.*, page 55.   Ploss, page 43.
[5] Hildebrandt.   *Ztschr. f. Ethn.*, 1878, vol. x., p. 394.
[6] Ploss, p. 42.

ity of Dr. Pollak, physician to the Shah, that the Persians are sometimes confined squatting on the ground, cross-legged, sometimes kneeling or sitting cross-legged; but it seems that the most popular position, and the one which appears to me to be far the most natural, and which bears a strong resemblance to our semi-recumbent position, whether in bed, or in the obstetric chair, or on the husband's lap, is the squatting position, as represented in the illustration of a woman with her legs apart, supporting herself upon her arms on a pile of three bricks, which she has placed on

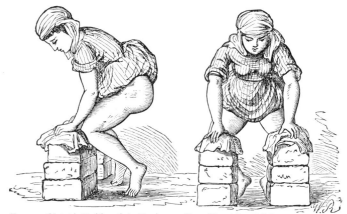

FIG. 10. Obstetric Position of the Persians. — From Ploss (after Pollak and Haentsche).

either side of her. In this position we have a remarkable illustration of the points which are developed in every perfect obstetrical position, namely, absolute relaxation of the muscles of the lower extremities and the pelvis, and separation of the limbs, in order to allow space for the passage of the child. The strain, if there be any, being upon the muscles of the arms and the chest.

The Zuñi women of New Mexico are delivered in this same position, which we may call a squatting one, and which is described to me as "half standing and half sitting;" an attendant supports the patient, and facilitates expulsion by pressing the abdomen from above downward.[1]

[1] T. F. Ealy, M. D.

In the neighboring Laguna Pueblo pretty much the same custom is followed. In the early stages of labor the patient stands, as she urinates, with her hands on her knees ; later, she stands up, supported by a woman on each side, or a rope is cast over a joist of the roof and allowed to hang down in a wide loop ; she puts her breast in the loop and holds on to the ascending ropes, her feet on the floor, in a half-sitting (squatting) posture, thus obtaining great expulsive force ; if tired and worn, she lies down. All these positions are assumed at the choice of the patient or the advice of her assistants, two to six in number.[1]

3. KNEELING.

The kneeling posture, like some other positions which appear to us peculiar, is a historical one. It is referred to in the Bible, as well as by the Roman poets. It was taught in ancient Rome, among the Arabs, and in Germany during the Middle Ages, and definite rules were laid down for the circumstances under which it should be resorted to. At this present day it is still, at times, adopted in the rural districts of our own States, and more frequently than we should suppose in our cities. It is that position which is, perhaps, most universal among our Indians, that is, among what we may call the blanket Indians, those who have not yet partially succumbed to the advances of eastern civilization. Some of our ablest obstetricians, Fellows of this Society, who have given me their opinions upon the kneeling posture in labor, differ in their views in regard to its advantages and disadvantages ; to one it seems physiologically correct, and appears most practically to favor the expulsion of the child, whilst it is frowned upon by another as liable to be followed by hemorrhage. We, however, do not hear of this as a frequent occurrence among the Indians, where the position is so common ; in fact, we neither hear of this nor any other accident consequent upon labor, not even of prolapse, which might be supposed to follow ; probably, because the position is only assumed during the

[1] John Menaul, U. S. Teacher.

advent of the more severe pains, and in the very last stage of labor.

If I may make a broad assertion, the kneeling posture seems most common among the red and yellow races ; our Indians mainly being delivered kneeling, with the body inclined forward ; whilst the Mongolians seem, as a rule, to retain the body more erect. I have classified the kneeling positions as follows : —

(*a.*) The body inclined forward.

(*b.*) This position overdone ; that is, with the body thrown

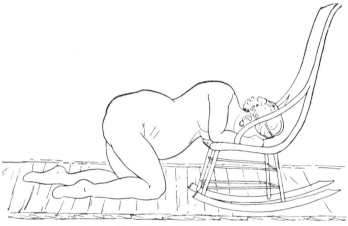

FIG. 11.—Southern Negress.

completely forward, the patient resting on the hands and knees, or knees and elbows.

(*c.*) The body erect or inclined backward, sometimes clinging to a rope.

(*d.*) Kneeling postures, where precise descriptions are lacking.

a. Kneeling, the Body inclined Forward.

It is the custom of most writers upon this subject to refer, like Legros,[1] Goodell, Ploss, and others, to the labor

[1] "De la position de la Femme pendant l'accouchement," *Gaz. des hôp.*, 1864, p. 133.

of Latona, whom Homer, in his hymn to Apollo, represents as being delivered whilst kneeling upon the soft meadow, clasping a palm tree. A somewhat more precise, though less poetic, description is given me of the labor of a Georgia negress : the physician being called in great haste, found his patient kneeling on a mat, placed on the floor, with her head and elbows resting on the seat of a rocking-chair, the thighs perpendicular, and the body nearly horizontal. The head had been born, but the shoulders resisted. Observing his patient for a few moments, he found that during the pains her body would move backward so that her buttocks rested upon her heels, whilst in the interval she would glide forward again, so that the thighs became perpendicular and the body horizontal. By his assistance, she was delivered of an enormously large child.[1]

In a previous labor she had been confined in a similar position, resting head and arms in the lap of her mistress ; precisely the same position which the squaws of the Umpgua tribe, in Oregon, are in the habit of assuming. Let us look in upon a scene of this kind.

The patient was found in a lodge, roughly constructed of lumber and drift-wood ; the place was packed to suffocation with men and women, the stifling odor from sweat and smoke and stench of whale oil, rendered the lodge unendurable for more than a few moments together. The parturient, situated in the centre of the place, was entirely naked excepting a covering by a dirty blanket, which was thrown across her loins. Her head and shoulders were supported in the lap of an old squaw, while her thighs were stoutly pressed against the pelvis by a squaw on each side, who were engaged in crowding the uterus downward in a brutal manner with their clenched fists, occasionally giving it a lateral motion ; another squaw sat between her knees, with her hands under the blanket, ready to receive the child when it came. The crowd in the lodge all the while kept up a deafening din by crying, shouting, pounding on tin vessels, and thumping up against the roof with poles ;

[1] Dr. H. F. Campbell.

occasionally the attendants at the patient's side would make passes over her in the mesmeric style, and spurt sprays of water upon her, after the fashion of Chinese laundrymen.[1]

Many of the Indian tribes follow this custom, the parturient woman assuming a kneeling position, head and arms resting in the lap of an attendant, or upon any convenient support: a stump, box, bed, or chair; so the tribes of the Quapaw Agency, the Peorias, Shawnees, Wyandots, Ottawas, and Senecas.[2]

The Indians of the Cattaraugus Reservation are delivered in the same way, assuming this position just before the expulsion of the child, whilst in the earlier stages they sit or walk about as they please.[3] So, also, the Clatsops of northwestern Oregon, who, however, retain the body more erect, as a young woman assistant stands behind the parturient and clasps her under the arms and around the breast, supporting the patient and forcibly holding her up.[4]

The whites equally resort to this position; thus I hear of its observance in the western and southwestern portions of Missouri. Dr. Willis P. King, of Sedalia, writes me that he has found quite a number of cases where the women desired, during the last part of the second stage, to get up and kneel by a chair; and he says that all the women who have been in the habit of being delivered in this way were Pennsylvanians, of the Pennsylvania German stock, or, at least, that the suggestion had come from a Pennsylvania woman. Since he has seen a woman flood almost to syncope after delivery in this position, he condemns it severely.

I am a little astonished to see this position mentioned as originating in this country among the Pennsylvania Germans, because the only reference that I can find to the kneeling posture among the Germans (and we cannot in reality call the Fins Germans) is by Holst,[5] who says that the Esthen, in difficult cases, seek to hasten delivery by assum-

---

[1] E. P. Vellum, M. D., Surgeon U. S. A.
[2] F. A. Bickford, M. D.   [3] A. D. Lake, M. D.
[4] J. Murray Dickson, M. D.
[5] *Beitr. z. Gynæk. u. Geburtsk.*, vol. ii., p. 114.

ing the kneeling posture, by suspending the woman, or placing her upon her husband's lap.   Among the early Scotch and English, however, it was more common, at least so it is told by Spence, in his "System of Midwifery," [1] who says that some women are inclined to be delivered kneeling down beside a chair or bed, leaning on it with their elbows or heads.   Irish, of the laboring classes in Massachusetts,

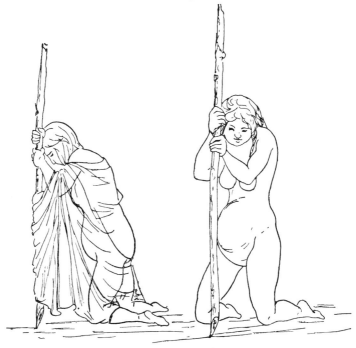

Fig. 12. — Blackfoot Squaw

are still occasionally delivered in this position, if left to themselves.[2]   The Armenians, and, in Greece, the Pelasgians, are delivered in the same position, kneeling, hands and arms resting on a chair, whilst the midwife is seated behind the patient to receive the child.[3]

Not having the convenience of a chair always at hand,

[1] Edinburgh, 1784, pp. 148–149.   [2] C. A. Wilcox, M. D.
[3] Dr. Damean George.   Ploss, p. 40.

but seeking instinctively to further labor by this same kneeling position, with the body inclined forward, the North American Indian seizes a staff or tent-pole. This is true of some Indians belonging to the Sioux Nation, — the Blackfeet, the lower and upper Yankton-ais, and Uncpapas.[1] In these tribes I am told that the parturient woman is generally assisted by an old squaw, the recognized midwife of the camp, or by a female relation. She assumes the kneeling posture, — knees apart, body inclined forward, hands resting upon a staff or *té-pee* pole, head resting on the arms. Sometimes the arms rest on a trunk, or other suitable object to lean upon. The staff referred to is known as the "Honpê," an instrument used for digging the Pomme-blanc, or wild Indian turnip, and may be regarded as the original support used during delivery. This posture is maintained during the expulsion. The same is true of the Caddo, Delaware, Kiowa, and Comanche Indians.[2] "The patient generally walks about the lodge during the first stage of labor, but as the second stage begins she assumes the kneeling position, and holds to a stake driven in the ground in front of her."

The same custom is observed among the Comanches and the Indians of the Unitah Valley, who, however, are not confined in their *té-pee* but in a temporary enclosure near by. The accompanying cut represents a Comanche squaw in labor, and in order that it may be fully understood I will give some of the details of this accouchement from the extremely interesting description of Major W. H. Forwood, Surgeon U. S. A., who was in attendance and kindly furnished the sketch: "A short distance outside the camp, and in the rear of the patient's family lodge, a shelter had been constructed of green boughs, six or seven feet high, by making holes in the hard ground with a wooden peg, and setting up brush or bushes, with the leaves on, around the circumference of a circle about eight feet in diameter. An

[1] Surgeon L. M. Maus, U. S. A., Fort Yates, D. T.

[2] Dr. L. L. McCabe, Physician to the Kiowa, Comanche, and Wachita Agency ; Maj. M. Barber, U. S. A.

entrance was provided by breaking the circle and overlapping the two unjoined ends; in a line outside the entrance

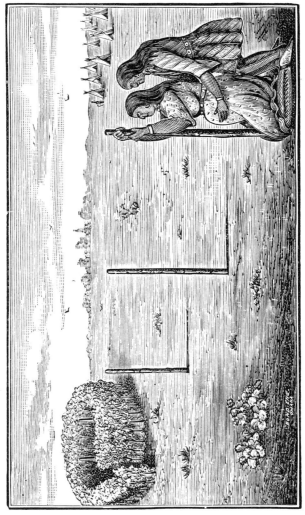

FIG. 13. Comanche Labor.

Sketch by Major W. H. Forwood, Surgeon U S. A

were three stakes, ten paces apart, set firmly upright in the ground, four feet high.

Inside the shelter were two rectangular excavations in the grass-covered soil, about twelve by sixteen inches, with a stake at one end of each ; in one of these holes was a hot stone, and in the other a little loose earth to receive any discharge that might take place from the bladder or bowels ; the ground about was strewn with a few aromatic herbs ; sometimes a lariat secured to a limb overhead may take the place of the stakes to hold to during a pain.

I found my patient walking with her assistant, a female relative, up and down the line of stakes outside the shelter, stooping now and then to kneel at the nearest stake and grasping it with both hands during a pain ; most of her time was spent in this way, outside the enclosure ; occasionally she would enter to kneel over the hot stones or loose earth. During each pain she knelt 'down close to one of the stakes, bringing the front of her feet and legs against the ground and her knees a little apart, the body bent forward, face turned down, or sometimes up, at the severest part of the pain, and the hands, one above the other, grasping the stake on about a level with the head. The assistant stood behind, astride of or between the patient's feet, and stooping over, passed her arms around the body until her hands were brought over the front and lower· part of the patient's abdomen ; in this position she performed several manipulations with the palms of her hands and fingers, while the pain lasted, such as rubbing, kneading, etc., but most frequently a quick jerking or shaking upward movement, something like that of shaking a pillow into its case. The patient never assumed a recumbent position, and the moment the placenta escaped she sprang up, buckled on a stout leather belt, mingled with the crowd and soon disappeared, without apparently·taking the slightest notice of her child."

The Indians of the Unitah Valley Agency, Utah, observe the same customs with this exception, that they keep a kettle of hot water, boiling, within the enclosure or " Wicke-up," of which the patient takes frequent and copious draughts during the labor, and as soon as the child is expelled she continues drinking freely of the hot water, rises to her feet, places a folded cloth to her abdomen, and leaning forward over a short stake, rests her body upon it, thus exerting considerable pressure over the hypogastric region, which is supposed to favor the expulsion of the placenta.[1]

The natives of New Zealand kneel down upon a mat, the knees about two feet apart, the hands resting on a tree or stick, or clutching some hard substance, while if help is needed, the arms are twined about the knees of an assistant in order to press them against the fundus of the womb.[2]

The Dakota woman assumes a kneeling position during labor, unless extreme weakness prevents; she supports herself by a post driven into the ground, or any convenient means of support; the recumbent position, they think, retards the progress of labor.[3]

The rather vague information to be obtained from the Cheyennes, Arapahoes, and Eastern Apaches was to the effect that the parturient woman, as among so many of the Indian tribes, retires to the bush, where, if the labor is a normal one, she is delivered without any assistance, the position assumed being upon her knees, occasionally a reclining one. Dr. C. P. Allen writes me concerning the Chippewas, from the White Earth Indian Agency, that, if the parturient is of the wild or blanket Indians, a quantity of dry grass is spread on the ground in the *té-pee*, or house, if they have any; a pole six to ten feet long and three to four inches in diameter is placed on the backs of chairs or fixed across one corner of the room about the height of a chair, behind which, with it across her chest, the woman rests on her knees during the pains, sitting down in the interval. Those who are partly civilized assume a somewhat similar position but use straw overlaid by quilts or blankets.

I would here call attention to the fact that the Chippewa woman seems to draw horizontally upon this cross-bar and

[1] Frank S. Bascom, M. D.

[2] *Brit. and For. Med.-chir. Rev.*, Lond., 1855, vol. xv., page 525. Hooker, *Journal of the Ethnological Society*, of London, 1869, page 69. Goodell, page 674.

[3] Dr. J. W. Cook, Yankton Agency.

not to rest herself, or raise herself, as do those Indians who support themselves by a staff or pole. An Indian interpreter, F. F. Gerard, who has spent some thirty years among the Indians, especially the Rees, Gros-Ventres, and Mandans, and has had a good deal of practice in their camps, writes me from Fort Abraham Lincoln, that, with the assistance of several women, the parturient is confined in a kneeling

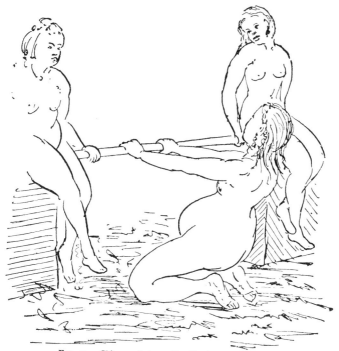

FIG 14.— Chippewa Labor. Kneeling inclined backwards.

posture, her head resting on her arms, which are crossed upon her bosom, and raised about fifteen inches from the ground : a large piece of skin is placed upon the ground or a blanket is used, and three or four inches of dirt are strewn upon the skin or blanket, then another piece of skin or blanket is placed over this for the woman to kneel upon, the head upon the edge of the bed. This position is assumed during every pain until the delivery takes place.

This is a kneeling position with the body so far inclined forward that it approaches the knee-hand, knee-chest, knee-elbow posture, to which we next come.

From a very instructive letter, recently received from Dr. N. Kauda, of Tokio, I see that the Japanese are not unfrequently delivered in a kneeling posture; the descrip-

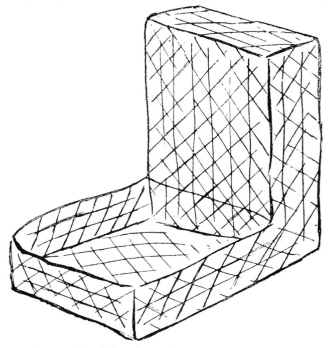

FIG. 15. — Framework formerly in use in Japan for the support of the parturient in a kneeling posture.

tion of the labor is as received from the mouth of one " ignorant of the modern laws of obstetrics." During labor and the expulsion of the child the woman is in a (sitting) kneeling posture, *i. e.*, the body supported on the tips of the toes and the knees ; the reason for this is to prevent the rush of blood to the head. The body is bent forward, and the patient supports herself by seizing hold of a midwife, who moreover assists by rubbing her abdomen. This is in case she can afford to call in two midwives, as a more skillful one is needed to take charge of the labor. As a rule the inferior assistant is dispensed with, and a framework about one foot and a half square is used as a convenient support for the patient to hold to.

Fifty years ago the patient was supported in her position and the labor conducted in a framework (Fig. 15), but now ordinary articles of bedding are piled up to support the back (Fig. 16), as seen in the figure which represents the posture just after delivery, and in this upright position

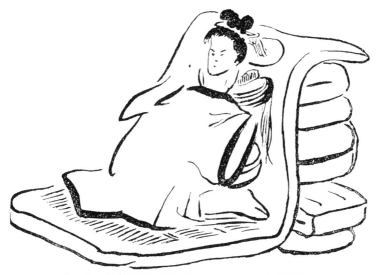

FIG. 16. — Sitting Posture of the Japanese; customary in Childbirth.

the patient remains for some three days, when gradually the prop is removed from behind her back until finally she is lying, as usual, with her head on but one pillow.

(b.) *Knee-Hand or Knee-Elbow Position.*

The knee-elbow position seems of old to have been recommended by the ablest obstetricians for very stout persons. Thus Soranus, and later the Arab, Jahiah Ebu Serapion, and Rhazes, who lived in the first half of the ninth century, advises the knee-elbow position under these circumstances ; so, also, later, among the Germans, Roesslin[1] tells us that this same treatment of fat women is found in the works of Hippocrates, Galen, Paul of Ægina,[2] Aetius,[3] and was used by most of the " modern ancients." Nor was it confined to remote times ; for in some portions of Russia, Greece, and Turkey women are yet confined in this way.

In 1779, Hopkins objected to the lateral position and urged that the position on the hands and knees was the best.[4] Denman was of opinion that "this posture is instinctively sought by unassisted women."[5] Whilst in 1791, that shrewd observer Charles White quoted Denman approvingly, and argued that the " knee-elbow position in natural labor prevented too great a pressure on the perineum."[6] According to Ramsbotham,[7] "the peasantry of Ireland placed themselves upon their hands and knees, and in Cornwall it is difficult to persuade the woman in labor to take any other posture than standing or on her knees." It is interesting to see how people carry these customs, which have been traditional among them for ages, across the seas.

We have seen the southern Negroes following the African ways, and the same may be observed among the Welsh, the Irish, and Germans ; thus, Dr. H. C. Yarrow tells me that he had a patient once, a Welsh woman, who insisted on crawling on hands and knees while the pains were progressing, and who informed him that in Wales women frequently assumed this position or were delivered sitting upon the laps of their husbands. Irish women, who, as I am informed by several correspondents,[8] are in this country delivered in the hand and knee position, assert that this is

---

[1] Goodell, page 675.
[2] Lib. iii., cap. lxii., 76.
[3] *De Conceptus et Partus Ratione,* cap. 22.
[4] *The Accoucheur's Vade Mecum.*
[5] *Archives of Midwifery,* London, 1792, part i., page 58.
[6] *Management of Pregnant Lying-in Women,* London, 1791, p. 104.
[7] Second edition, page 122.
[8] Dr. Baldwin, of Columbus, Ohio.

frequently resorted to by women of their nationality abroad. Some of our ablest obstetricians consider the knee-elbow position a decidedly favorable one for version. Dr. Campbell, of Augusta, had a most successful case of this kind which he described and which should have been published in the "Transactions" of this Society, but by some accident was mislaid; he seems to think that when the woman is in labor the contents of the pelvic cavity are, by this position, relaxed in a most remarkable manner, making it very favorable for version. Dr. Parvin of Indianapolis has published a similar case, which has deservedly excited attention. These learned gentlemen, however, need not claim any credit to themselves, as the untutored redskin now does, and probably has for centuries done, the same thing. The Cheyenne and Arapahoe squaws, who usually assume the dorsal decubitus, seek a change of position in case of protracted labor, and not unfrequently the knee-elbow position to facilitate or hasten labor.[1]

Major Charles R. Greenleaf, surgeon U. S. A., informs me that the Nez-Percés and Gros-Ventres women, who in ordinary labor are confined in a stooping posture, in cases where labor is protracted assume the knee-elbow position, whilst the patient's abdomen is encircled by a broad belt, upon which force is exerted by assistants, placed on either side of the patient, who scrupulously direct this force backwards and downwards during pains. The doctor himself witnessed such a case of protracted labor in a Gros-Ventre squaw, a primipara, who assumed the ordinary knee-elbow position and about whose abdomen a belt, often called the "squaw-belt," was placed.

The pressure exercised by the "squaw-belt" among the Gros Ventre Indians is supplied by the pillow among the Creeks, and the encircling arms of an assistant among the Kootenais, whose labors are conducted in a most peculiar fashion, the parturient taking the knee-elbow position; she is on her knees, the face touching the ground; hands, one above the other, grasping a pole planted in the ground,

[1] J. H. Bannister, M. D.

head touching the hands ; legs apart. A male assistant stands astraddle of the patient, over her buttocks, his hands clasped around her waist ; during each pain he pulls, thus making pressure on the abdomen.[1]

The Modocs, who as yet have assumed but few of the customs of civilized life, are always delivered in this position ; their method is as peculiar as it is instructive, and is worthy our most careful consideration ; they maintain a curved position, lying on the side, until the labor is nearly completed, when they assume the position on their knees and hands, which is continued until the child is born.[2]

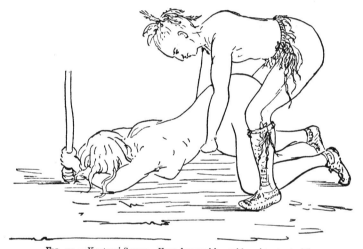

FIG. 17. — Kootenai Squaw.   Knee-face position, with assistant astraddle.

Experience has evidently taught them that these different positions assumed during various stages of labor would make it progress most rapidly, with least pain to themselves.

In ordinary cases the Creeks assume what we might call an overdone knee-chest position ; they are delivered lying on face and chest, and hence I have classed them as horizontally recumbent.

[1] E. L. Morgan, M. D.
[2] F. A. Bickford, M. D., Quapaw Agency.

(*c.*) *Kneeling, with the body erect, inclined backward, or partially suspended.*

This, like other of those apparently peculiar positions which are fast yielding to the westward march of civilization and scientific medicine, was at one time not unusual in our States, and I will cite the early experience of Dr. Reamy in Ohio as characteristic of the practice thirty years ago; he says : " I have found in my practice ten or twelve different women, who had frequently borne children before, who insisted, with a perseverance and determination that I dared not resist, in being out upon the floor, down upon their knees, leaning backward so that the buttocks almost touched the heels. The husband knelt behind the wife, with his arms around her, his broad strong hands acting as a pad for the abdomen, and making pressure during pains — à la Crédé — her shoulders resting against the man's chest. These women insisted that this was the only position in which they could be comfortably and successfully delivered." The same position, practically, is found among the Papagos. Among these Indians, " the position of the squaw, from the time the labor pains commence until the expulsion of the fetus and placenta, is a kneeling one, with the knees sufficiently spread to furnish comfortable lateral support to the body, which is erect. In the interval between the pains she is allowed to move about according to her inclination. In ordinary labors two women assist her. One of them places herself in a kneeling position behind the parturient woman, and with one knee pressing firmly in the lumbar region, she grasps with both hands the body of the patient immediately under the ribs in front. The other assistant places herself in a kneeling position in front of the woman, and with the palms of both hands rubs the abdominal wall down from the spine of the ilium to the pubes. It is interesting to note that they seem to appreciate the necessity and advisability of time and patience with primiparæ, as they do not resort to the same degree of pressure and friction which they employ in assisting multiparæ.[1]

[1] J. O. Skinner, M. D., Surgeon U. S. A., Fort Lowell, A. T.

The Yuma Indians vary this position somewhat.[1] The parturient woman is assisted by two others of long experience in the business. One of these kneels behind her, supporting her body in nearly an upright position, her arms passing under those of the patient and pressing or smoothing down the abdomen. The other assistant squats in front, between the feet of the patient, with her ankles crossed, and her shins pressed against those of the parturient woman, whilst she holds her by the hands or wrists. The posture of the patient is, therefore, with the shoulders high, the legs and thighs strongly flexed and abducted, which position is retained until the expulsion of the placenta. No bandage is used.

The Upper Klamath and nearly related Modocs of Oregon are usually delivered in a small lodge some distance away from the other houses. The parturient also assumes a kneeling position, supported by one old squaw, whilst another keeps kneading and rubbing her abdomen. Sometimes she varies her posture by sitting and pressing her feet against some support, while she bears down. If labor is tedious, they often sit over warm stones moistened with water, or, in other words, take a steam bath to relax the system. They also steam themselves occasionally for several days after the birth of the child.[2]

Precisely this same position is found among many of the Mongolians, especially the Tartars, if we may accept the authority of Hureau de Villeneuve.[3] The parturient moves about during the early pains, sometimes standing with her hands above her head, but as soon as the bearing-down pains begin she assumes the kneeling position last described, almost erect, supporting her body upon the hands, which rest upon the separated knees or thighs; the assistant behind supports her by seizing her under the arms, whilst the midwife rests upon one knee in front of the pa-

---

[1] Surgeon J. K. Carson, U. S. A.

[2] James S. Dennison, M. D.

[3] *De l'accouchement dans la race jaune*, Paris, 1863, p. 32; Ploss, p. 40.

tient. The author seems to think that the advantages of this position are greater than its disadvantages, that the abdominal muscles come more freely into play, and that there is less danger of rupture of the perineum, as the head of the child, following the pelvic axis, tends by its own weight towards the vaginal orifice, and not towards the perineum, which in this way escapes the pressure necessarily bearing upon it in any other position. Prolapse is not known among them. While writing this my attention is called to a circular just received, giving the titles of papers entered to be read before the subsection of Anthropology, at the coming meeting of the American Association for the Advancement of Sciences, to be held in Boston, August, 1880. I find that a paper is announced entitled, "Parturition: Kneeling Posture as practiced by the Women of the Mound Builders and Stone Grave Races," by Rev. C. Foster Williams of Ashwood, Maury Co., Tenn. In answer to an inquiry, Mr. Williams states that he has in his collection of Mound Builder relics an earthen vessel, which he supposes to represent a woman in labor: the right knee on the ground, with the right hand resting on that knee; the left foot on the ground, the left hand resting on the left knee.[1] Although sorry to disabuse Mr. Williams of his belief, I must state that this position cannot possibly be assumed by a parturient woman, as the muscles would not be relaxed, and proper space would not be given for the passage of the child.

My attention once called to the subject, I examined my own collection, and found in it two images representing a woman in the erect kneeling posture, the knees somewhat separated, the hands resting upon the knees or thighs in precisely the same position as that assumed by the Mongolians, and probably the Yumas. It is not unlikely that these figures represent parturient women, and it is highly probable that the mythical Mound Builders, be they predecessors of our Indians, or older tribes of the same stock,

---

[1] This position is advocated by Herr V. Ludwig as the most favorable one for the first stage of labor.

were delivered of their young in the same position as the red squaws of the present day. Hence we may take the testimony of these vessels, relics of a former civilization, that the position assumed by the Mound Builder race in parturition was the erect kneeling one.

The kneeling, partially suspended, position is found among the Indians and lower classes of Mexicans in the neighborhood of San Luis Potosi. The labor is conducted in the following way : a round stick of pine wood, eighteen or

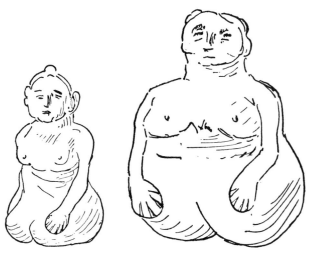

FIG. 16.—Images from the Period of the Mound Builders   From the Burial Mounds of
Missouri.

twenty feet long, and half a foot in diameter, is placed against the head of the bed or the wall, its other end resting upon the floor at an angle of about forty-five degrees; to this beam a cord is tied, knotted at one end, and covered with soft cloths. The parturient woman kneels upon a sheep-skin spread upon the floor, seizes the knotted end of the cord in her hands, and is delivered in a kneeling, semi-suspended position, by the *partera* or midwife.[1] Dr. Barroeta says also that prolapse and displacement of the uterus are not uncommon, and does not know why they are

---

[1] Dr. G. Barroeta.

not still more frequent. From other sources I also hear that the lower orders of Spanish women nearly always take the kneeling position, and, as Dr. Coates writes me from Pueblo, Col., " if the placenta is tardy they always drink a cupful of soapsuds, which produces vomiting, followed by the immediate expulsion of the afterbirth."

The lower classes of Northern Mexico speak the Spanish language and profess the Catholic faith, but in all other respects are Indians, and retain many Aztec customs ; so

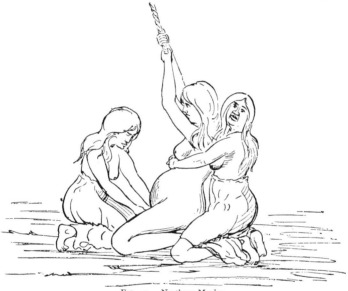

Fig 19.— Northern Mexico.

the accouchement, which is described to me by Surgeon George W. Adair, U. S. A., precisely as we have seen it among the Indians near San Luis Potosi, the patient kneeling, grasping a rope pendent from the ceiling, and assisted by *tendera* and *partera*, " the tendera fixing the knees, and holding the upper portion of the trunk, as in a vice, pulls the pelvis forward, hinged as it is upon the acetabulum, and thus overcomes the dip of the plane of the superior strait, and straightens the passage with greater efficacy and certainty."

The American Indians on the frontier of Mexico follow the same traditional method of delivery, hanging on a rope suspended from a rafter, with the knees bent and just off the ground. The rope, which is wrapped with cloths or towels so as to make it softer, usually hangs at the edge of the bed, so that the patient can stand on her feet or sit or

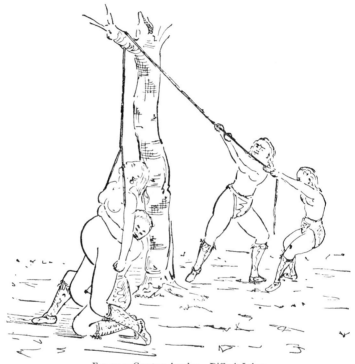

Fig. 20. — Coyotero Apaches. Difficult Labor.

recline on the bed during the intervals between the pains. The partera introduces her hand and presses on the perineum, not making a steady pressure, but during the entire time of the pain she jolts the patient up and down, imagining that she is shaking the child out.[1]

The Coyotero Apaches place the parturient in a similar position, suspending her a good deal more, in difficult cases,

[1] C. M. Harrison, M. D.

if she does not succeed in expelling the child in the squatting posture customary among them. "A rope or lariat is tied around the woman's chest just beneath her arms, and the other end thrown over a stout limb of an adjacent tree, while two or three squaws draw upon this until the woman's knees barely touch the ground; others, generally two, encircle the body with their arms, and 'strip' down with considerable force, a kind of 'all pull together,' as it were. This energetic manœuvre generally suffices for prompt uterine work." [1]

The Santee Indians are almost invariably delivered in a kneeling posture on the floor, with a bench or chair in front of them upon which they rest their arms, while sometimes they have a rope attached above by which they partially suspend themselves, just as the Mexican Indians and half-breeds do.[2]

(*d.*) *Kneeling Postures, where Precise Description is Lacking.*

Unfortunately, Dr. Ploss, in his valuable and interesting work, has failed to define precisely the positions assumed, and, as I have been unable to refer to the authorities myself, I will take the liberty of stating in a general way, upon the authority of Dr. Ploss, that the kneeling posture is assumed occasionally, at least, by women in labor in Nicaragua,[3] in Finland,[4] in modern Greece,[5] in Kamtschatka, in eastern Asia; and, if we go back to the Middle Ages, among the Abyssinians,[6] a people who originally came from Asia, where, as we have already said, among the yellow races the kneeling posture is a common one; also, under certain circumstances, in Rome; among the Arabs and Germans in the Middle Ages. Finally, in ancient times, among the Pelasgians, if some Greek authors are correctly translated.

If I may be permitted to refer to the somewhat vague

[1] Walter Reed, M. D., Surgeon U. S. A.

[2] Dr. George W. Ira.

[3] W. Marr, *Reise nach Central Amerika*, Hamburg, 1863, vol. i., p. 275.

[4] Holst.   [5] Prof. George.   [6] J. Ludolf, 1681.

statements in the Bible, we find in 1 Samuel, iv. 19, "Phineas' wife bowed herself and travailed, for her pains came upon her." This passage, I am informed, is commonly rendered by learned commentators as kneeling; Gesenius, in his Hebrew Lexicon, so understands the word. In Job, iii. 12, "Why did the knees prevent me," the Latin word being *prevenio,* to go before; as if Job had said, "Why did not the knees of my mother remain rigid and stiff, and I strangle in birth." The whole passage sustains this idea of kneeling.[1]

4. SEMI-RECUMBENT.

The semi-recumbent positions are by far the most frequent among the ancients, especially among the more civilized people of olden times, and among the savage races of the present day. The same position of the body is assumed by various races in very different ways, there being apparently no resemblance in the method of delivery, whilst it appears, upon more careful study, that the position of the body, the inclination of the trunk and the pelvic axis, together with the relaxed position of the thighs, is almost identical, the same end being accomplished in ways very different, peculiar to each people, and in keeping with their surroundings. Thus, the simplest of the semi-recumbent positions, which is upon a par with the customs of the rudest African races, is sitting upon the ground, upon a stone or rude cushion, with the body inclined backward, leaning against an assistant, a tree, or some other object. A marked progress is achieved, when we find the parturient woman seated in the lap of an assistant reclining against his chest, a position which reaches its greatest perfection in the obstetric chair. As the next step, I regard the dorsal decubitus, a position modified according to the circumstances of the people. In the wilds of Africa, and in the interior of our western country, the patient finds her couch upon the floor, propped up against some staves of wood or a pile of grass, whilst in the lying-in chamber of the civilized peo-

[1] C. Foster Williams.

ple we find the same position assumed upon the bed, and this I look upon as the perfection of obstetric positions, the easiest, most comfortable, and advantageous.

(*a.*) *Sitting Semi-recumbent on the Ground, upon a Stone, or Stool.*

Among our Indians we find that the Otoes, Missouris, Omahas, Iowas, and nearly related tribes assume the sitting posture, the legs widely separated ; but as the crisis supervenes, the patient raises herself somewhat by a rope suspended above, thus attaining an inclined, semi-recumbent position.[1] The Wakah squaw assumes a sitting posture, on the floor of the lodge, with nothing but an Indian mat under her. As soon as the labor pains come on her feet are drawn up close to the buttocks, and the legs flexed ; this position is maintained until after the birth of the child and the expulsion of the placenta.[2]

The women of the Skokomish Agency, W. T., sit down with a pillow or roll of blankets resting against the perineum ; one squaw supports the back, while another receives the child. This position is a slightly recumbent one, the buttocks resting on the pillow or roll of blankets.[3] The Confederated tribes of the Flatheads, Pend d'Oreilles, and Kootenais, follow a similar custom : a small box, or a piece of wood, six or eight inches high, covered with old pieces of blanket or buffalo robes, is the seat upon which the sick woman is placed ; her legs are separated and flexed so that the heels almost come in contact with the seat. She is retained in that position by two assistants who hold her by the arms, and sometimes a third one stands behind and presses upon her shoulders, and in this position the child is expelled.[4]

Though apparently uncomfortable and inconvenient, and rare among the the American Indians, the Kaffirs univer-

[1] Dr. W. C. Botener, Otoe Agency, Nebraska.
[2] J. N. Powers, M. D., Neah Bay Agency, W. T.
[3] J. W. Givens, M. D.
[4] L. H. Choquette, M. D.

sally adopt this obstetric position, sitting with the heels
drawn up to the buttocks, the shoulders generally resting
against one of the poles supporting the roof of the hut, or
against some one of the female friends, who are present in
full force.

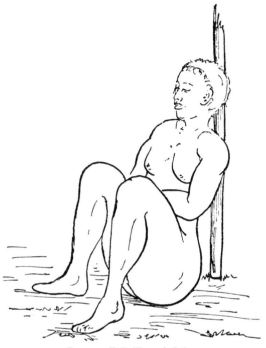

FIG. 21. — Kaffir Woman in Labor.

A somewhat similar position in labor seems to be followed in Germany by Russian emigrants who came there
in 1858 (Prussian Pomerania). They, however, do not raise
the shoulders so much. Dr. C. J. Egan, who makes this
statement,[1] adds : " The Kaffir position is a very good one,
and the woman has full power to bear down and assist her
pains. Of course, in this position, no support can be given
to the perineum by the hand of the attendant, but I am
much inclined to think that some very useful support is

[1] *Midwifery Notes from British Kaffraria, in South Africa.*

given the perineum from its resting on the firm floor of the hut, and the sudden passage of the child's head is thereby prevented."

The Kaffir and the Indian woman sit upon the ground, whilst the somewhat more advanced half-breed, as she is often found in Southern California and New Mexico, seats herself upon a chair, and during the pains, in the same way as her Indian sister, grasps a rope suspended from the ceiling above ; but, when tired out in this position, she is often found kneeling upon the ground.[1] A white sister involuntarily testifies to the efficiency of this position, at least under certain conditions, — a primipara who had been in labor for two days and was confined on the third, in a sitting posture, the pains ceasing entirely whenever she assumed a recumbent position ; of this the observing attendant, Dr. Von Mansfelde, of Ashland, Neb., assured himself. In order to satisfy himself that it was not the whim of a parturient woman, he placed her on the bed, on her side and back, several times, but the hand placed upon the fundus showed complete relaxation; no sign of contraction. When replaced in the sitting posture the pains readily returned, and were very effective, the woman being delivered within two hours after dilatation of the os.

The Arab woman is seated on two flat stones, or, more properly, her buttocks are slightly supported upon two flat stones, whilst during each pain she partially raises herself by a rope which is suspended from the centre-pole of the tent. Two assistants seize the parturient woman under the shoulders, and she herself, during the pain, raises herself by the rope ; they aid this motion, partially suspend her, shaking her well, as the miller does his sack of flour when he empties it, and then, as the pains cease, they drop her back upon the stones. This, at least, was the practice witnessed in several cases in 1858 by Dr. Goguel,[2] in one instance,

---

[1] King, *Am. J. Sc.*, April, 1853, p. 891.
[2] "Accouchement chez les Hebreux et les Arabes," *Gaz. hebd. de méd.*, No. 23.

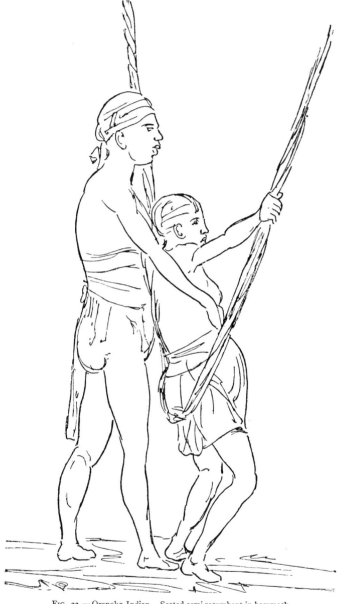

Fɪɢ. 22. — Oronoko Indian.   Seated semi-recumbent in hammock

the patient being the wife of a sheik. In Massana, upon the Red Sea, the woman of the lower classes sits, in the same way, upon a flat stone, reclining against some convenient support, or held in the arms of a friend. The natives of the Antilles not unfrequently assume a sitting, semi-recumbent position. In some portions of South America, where hammocks serve so many purposes, for instance, among the Indians of the Oronoko and Guiana, the parturient woman is delivered while seated upon the hammock, which is rolled almost into a rope. The assistant stands behind to support the patient, whilst the midwife, often a very skillful woman, is seated in front, and remains to fulfill her office.[1]

A most admirable position, typically semi-recumbent, was customary in Greece and her provinces 2,200 years ago, as is proven by that interesting group, representing a labor just completed, which was discovered by General di Cesnola during his researches in Cyprus ; we, moreover, have the same undeniable evidence that this marble group faithfully represents the obstetric position in Cyprus twenty-two centuries ago as we have of the correctness of the Peruvian posture at the time of the Inkas, as pictured upon the funeral urn. The native Peruvians of the present day are still confined whilst seated upon the husband's lap ; and the Cypriote midwife of to-day still places her patient in the semi-recumbent position upon a low stool which she carries about with her.

In response to my inquiries, General di Cesnola kindly furnished me with the following most valuable information. He says : " The group was found among the *débris* of the temple at Golgoi, in 1871, and is of the best Greek epoch, say 400 B. C. The chair on which the woman is reclining, is Cypriote, and was probably used also in Greece at that period ; the modern Cypriote midwives possess similar low chairs, which they carry with them when going to attend a child-birth, and I have myself seen the circumstances as shown in that group, which faithfully represents the partu-

[1] Dr. George W. Barr.

rition scene of to-day. An assistant of the midwife's is
kneeling behind the patient, holding her head upon her
shoulder ; the midwife, who is seated upon a very low stool
in front of the parturient and between her separated legs,
has just extracted the child which she has on her arms.
The exhausted woman, seated in a semi-recumbent position
on a low stool, still has her legs wide apart, but has been
covered with a blanket and is left to rest for a few minutes

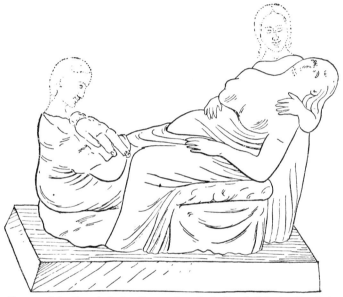

FIG. 23.— Labor Scene in Ancient Greece.   Group in the Cesnola Collection, New York

previous to being replaced in her bed. . . . . The chairs
which I have seen, and especially the one which the midwife of Larnaca brought to the house of our friend, had no
pillows, but two arms ; and the seat, though not perforated,
had a peculiar shape, with a ridge in the centre, evidently
made for the purpose of keeping the legs apart as much as
possible."

  Although Cyprus was held at various times by Pheni-
cians, Assyrians, Egyptians, Persians, and Romans, this
much mutilated group so unmistakably bears the imprint

of Greek art that we must look upon it as representing the custom of those people and those of Cyprus during the Greek period, and well representing it, for the position of the parturient is an admirable one, unmistakably seated, semi-recumbent, upon a low stool, which cannot be termed an obstetric chair, as is done in the description of the group in the "Transactions of the Edinburgh Obstetrical Society."[1] Great importance is attached to it by the author of that paper, as demonstrating the antiquity of the obstetric chair, but the fallacy of this view is already well proven by the criticism of Seligman in Virchow's "Jahresbericht."

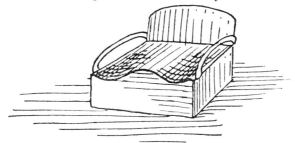

Fig. 24.—Modern Cypriote Midwife's Chair.

In southern India the patient walks about during the earlier stages of labor, then sits upon the ground with the thighs well separated, the back supported by an assistant, whilst the delivery itself is finally accomplished while lying upon the ground.[2]

(b.) *Sitting on the Lap or between the Thighs of an Assistant who is seated on a Chair or on the Floor.*

I look upon this position as identical with that on the obstretric chair, although more simple and more ancient ; and I believe that it will be apparent to every one, if the relative positions are considered, that the obstetric chair is merely an imitation of the more pliable and sensitive support afforded by the husband or assistant, who is himself made to suffer whilst holding the parturient woman during

---

[1] 1878, vol. iv., p. 50.
[2] Shortt, *Edinb. M. J.*, Dec., 1864, p. 554.

the tedious hours of labor. I am heartily in accord with the statement of Rigby, although seriously questioned by Ploss, that, "as far as we may rely upon the meagre records which history gives us upon this subject, among the more civilized people of antiquity the semi-recumbent sitting posture was by far the most common. In proof of this I will again refer to the oft-mentioned funeral urn which so vividly pictures the position of patient, husband, and nurse in the lying-in chamber during the moment of the greatest trial, during the expulsion of the child. The patient is seated in the lap of an assistant. I can hardly say whether this is the husband or a female assistant, whether it is a male or female figure; at all events she is seated in the lap of a person whose arms encircle her waist, the hands pressing firmly upon the fundus of the uterus. The midwife is seated upon a low stool, between the separated legs of the patient, and is just in the act of receiving the head of the new-born child. This vessel, called *Huaco*, represents a parturient scene precisely as it is still enacted among the descendants of the Incas to this day, and Dr. Coates assures me that he has, during his stay in Peru, not unfrequently acted accoucheur, the woman always taking this position with the husband behind. Upon that entire coast of South America the inhabitants seem faithfully to adhere to the customs of their ancestors, and no better proof can be found of the correctness of the representation of the labor scene depicted upon this vessel than the above statement of Dr. Coates, and of other physicians, the most interesting of which is perhaps one by Dr. Ruschenberger,[1] who, whilst in Colina, in Chili, in 1823, was called to a case of placenta previa and found a lady, a lady of rank by the way, with her feet near the foot of the bed, the knees drawn up, reclining against her husband, a rather short corpulent man, who was sitting in the middle of the bed wearing his riding cap, booted and spurred, with the legs extended on each side of her and his hands clasped in front of her chest to afford support. The antiquity of this position is also proven by a passage in

[1] *Am. J. Obst.*, Oct., 1879, p. 737.

Genesis (xxx. 3), which says that the Hebrew women were confined upon the lap of a female assistant.[1] In ancient Rome this position was assumed in cases either of urgent necessity, or among the poor where the obstetric chair was not to be had. Moschion teaches his readers to help themselves in this way and it seems that these teachings, revived in Italy by Joannis Michaelis of Savonarola,[2] finally found their way into Germany. In France, also, an author like De

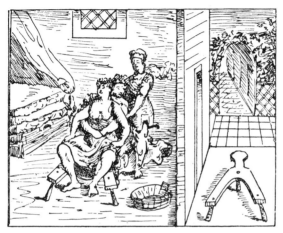

FIG. 25. — The Scientific Posture advocated in the 16th century. From Joannis Michaelis Savonarola, 1547.

La Motte[3] became a warm advocate of this position. Joannis Michaelis highly lauds a very low three-legged stool which serves as a seat for the assistant in whose lap the patient reclines ; he speaks of it as being of great antiquity, and much esteemed by the ancient Greeks. The assistant stands behind, on a rounded knob, supporting the patient, who is seated in front, upon the forked portion of the stool. At a comparatively late period a similar method of delivery was adopted among the modern Greeks.[4] The parturient

[1] Kotelmann, *Die Geburtsh. bei den alten Hebræern*, Marburg, 1876.

[2] *Practica major. Venetiis*, 1547, p. 280.

[3] *Traité*, 1721, liv. ii., chap. 12.

[4] W. Eton, *Schilderungen des türkischen Reiches ger.*, by Bergkt. Leipzig, 1805, page 144. Moreau, *Natur-gesch. des Weibes*, ii., page 194.

woman being seated upon a kind of tripod, behind her upon a somewhat higher stool sits an ·assistant whose arms are clasped over the fundus of the womb whilst the midwife is seated in front. I regard these positions as in the lap of an assistant and can certainly not look upon a simple stool, as it was probably found in any kitchen at the time, as an obstetric chair, but from that, most unquestionably, the obstetric chair takes its origin, and a very pointed statement to this effect is made by Dr. Metzler,[1] who in the early part of this century found an obstetric chair in some remote village where he little expected to see it, which had been constructed by a carpenter who had neither seen an obstetric chair nor heard of one ; but his wife had found her labor so easy, while sitting upon his lap, his legs separated, that he soon obtained a reputation in his native village, so that finally not a woman in the place would be confined in any other way than upon this good man's lap ; this he soon found so irksome that he constructed this chair, and, in his endeavors to copy the position assumed by himself, a very fair obstetric chair resulted.[2]   The above also seems to verify the statement that certain persons seem especially fitted, and acquire a reputation for such work ; in Holland they were a regular convenience at every labor, and were known as " shootsteers ; " but not only here and there in Germany, in France or Holland, but also among the early Scotch, Welsh, and English was this position frequently resorted to, and we need not be astonished to see this same custom in our own country.

We have seen how the modern Peruvians still follow the ways of the Incas, and so the descendants of these Germans, Welsh, or Scotch have not forgotten the habits of their ancestors, although they have crossed the seas and have mingled with a more enlightened civilization. It may surprise some of our city practitioners of to-day, who see little of the country population, and especially those who have not practised in rural districts years ago, that in our

---

[1] *Jenaisches Archiv. f. Geburtsh.*
[2] See Fig. 30.

own States women are confined sitting upon the lap of the husband or an assistant; this was, of course, much more frequent thirty years ago than it is now, but I still hear of it in many of our States, especially in southern Ohio, Pennsylvania, southwestern Missouri, Georgia, and the mountain regions of Virginia.

A graphic description of obstetric practice in the rural districts of Ohio is given me by Dr. E. B. Stevens of Lebanon, Ohio, and embodies all that has been written me from other States. To quote his own words: "When I commenced to practise, a good many years ago, the almost universal habit of confinement throughout the regions of south-

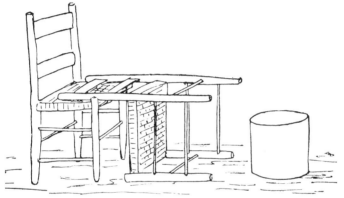

FIG. 26. — The Obstetric Couch.

ern Ohio was about as follows: two old-fashioned, straight-backed, slip-bottom chairs made the lounge, one chair erect the other turned down; a few old comforters upon this framework completed a very comfortable couch; the husband took his seat first, astride, the wife reclining in his arms, where she remained until labor was completed, unless there was much delay, in which case the patient was walked about or assumed any other position as dictated by fancy or impulse; the position of the accoucheur was upon an inverted half-bushel measure, so placed that he sat just between the limbs of the patient. Labor completed the soiled clothes were changed and the patient was placed in bed.

This position was certainly not a bad one for all parties with
the exception of the husband, who, in tedious cases, suffered
rather severely ; but then this little tax on his affectionate
nature was, in those days, considered the very least return
he could make for the mischief he had occasioned."

I have been told of this position in so many different
parts of this country that it would be superfluous to refer
to individual statements ; it is found in Pennsylvania, and
among Pennsylvania emigrants in southwestern Missouri,

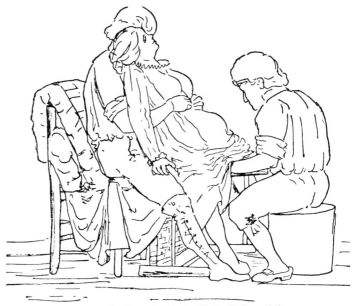

FIG. 27. — Semi-recumbent in the Husband's Lap. Ohio.

the position being practically the same, but differing somewhat in the details : thus, three chairs are placed in the
form of a triangle, facing towards a common centre ; the
husband takes his seat in one of these, and has a sheet,
or broad towel, or any cloth heavy enough, bound around
his thighs, leaving the knees about six inches apart. This
cloth serves as a seat for the parturient, and prevents the
husband's legs from spreading apart when tired by the long
continued strain ; the patient puts her feet on the rounds

of two other chairs, while a woman, seated in each of them, takes one of the patient's hands and supports the knee next to hers.

A professional friend in this State, who, like many other practitioners, tells me that the first patient he ever delivered was confined in this position, says that since then he has delivered quite a number of women in this way, and thinks it a great help in cases where the head constantly retreats after the pain ceases ; in the rural districts of Georgia both negro and white women, now and then, still

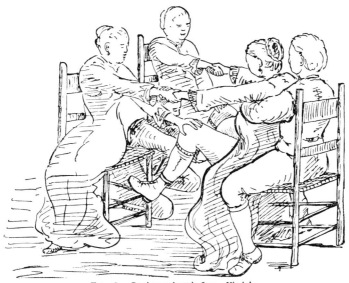

Fig. 28. — Semi-recumbent in Lap. Virginia.

follow this custom ; so, also, in Virginia. A very minute description of such a labor in the mountain districts of northwest Virginia, in the first third of this century, is given in the "New Orleans Medical and Surgical Journal" for 1860.[1] It is not surprising to see the white man thus patiently assisting his wife in the hour of her trial ; but it does seem somewhat strange that we should find this position, and the laborious duty imposed by it, undertaken by

[1] Dr. Dowler, *Position in Parturition*, p. 490.

our red brethren, as the Indian braves are usually so averse to work ; but I must say that it is only now and then, among the Utes and the Pueblos in Mexico, that this occurs, and they possibly have copied the Mexicans.

The Indians, and lower class of Mexicans in the vicinity of San Luis Potosi, are confined either in a kneeling position partially suspended, or sitting upon the floor. If confined in the latter position, the accouchée sits on a sheepskin on the floor, between the legs of one of the assistants, the *tenedora*, or holder, who is seated on a little cushion, and serves as a support to the patient, her thighs pressing against the patient's hips, and her arms encircling her waist, the hands clasped 'just above the fundus of the distended uterus, so that she can follow the child in its descent, and exert a gradual but strong compression ; the *partera*, of course, takes her position in front of the patient. Sometimes, in a tedious labor, this awkward posture is retained for one or two days, with not a little suffering to the *tenedora* as well as the patient.[1]

The custom of the Sandwich Islanders varies very little from this, and it is a matter of some interest to note their habits, as these islands, two thousand miles west of San Francisco, were entirely unknown one hundred years ago, and even fifty years ago were perfectly barbarous ; it is important to us, more especially as they still retain, in a great measure, their crude ideas and practices. Very interesting statements as to the obstetric practices in these islands are made by Dr. Charles H. Wetmore,[2] who has had a professional experience of twenty-two years upon Hawaii. When the labor is fairly commencing, the patient assumes a sitting posture upon a hard pillow or stone, her husband, or some intimate male or female friend, kneeling behind her, whose duty it is to clasp her above the abdomen in such a way that he can press down with considerable force upon the uterus and its contents, never relaxing this grasp to allow the fetus to recede. The accoucheur's position is in front ; she has little to do but to receive the child. Pre-

[1] Dr. G. Barroeta.   [2] *Buffalo M. & S. J.*, 1872–73, vol. xii., p. 90.

cisely the same custom prevails among the Andamanese, on the coast of India,[1] the only difference being that the patient and supporting husband are seated upon the ground. So, also, the Bedouins,[2] the child, however, being caught in a sieve, which is held by an assistant.

I have repeatedly had occasion to refer to the nomadic and barbarous tribes of Asia, as they have so successfully

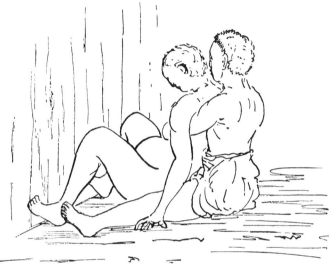

FIG. 29.—Andamanese Labor Scene.

resisted the encroachments and innovations of civilization, and among them many of these, to us peculiar positions, are still retained by parturient women ; but, like the Indian brave, the Asiatic warrior is little inclined to assist his suffering partner ; only among the Kalmucks is the parturient woman delivered in the lap of an assistant. The patient is seated upon the knees of a vigorous young man, who also exercises considerable pressure upon the abdomen by the hands which encircle the woman's waist.[3]   It seems pecul-

---

[1] " Jagor uber die Andamanesen oder Micopies," *Zeitschr. f. Ethnologie,* 1877, p. 51.

[2] Mayeaux, *The Bedouins,* chap. iii., p. 176.

[3] R. Krebel, *Volksmedic,* etc., p. 55; H. Meyerson, *Med. Ztg. Russlands,* 1860, xxiv., page 189 ; Ploss, 36.

iar that young men should, among some people, be chosen
for this office; here he serves as an obstetric chair, and
among the Brulé-Sioux a young warrior serves as a support for the parturient squaw, who suspends herself from
his neck ; only the Japanese see that the physician is an
aged male, in case that these positions are assumed for obstetric purposes.

(c). The Obstetric Chair.

The positions we have so far considered have been almost

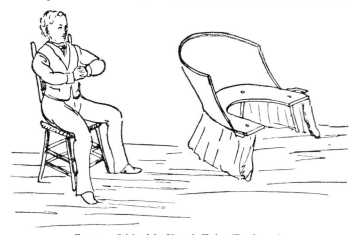

Fig. 30. — Origin of the Obstetric Chair. (Engelmann.)

·altogether such as required no artificial assistance and were
instinctively assumed.

With the advance of the obstetric art, the support given
the parturient woman by the bone and muscle of her kin,
by husband or tenedora, was replaced by a form of wood;
the thighs upon which she sat, the chest against which she
rested, were replaced by the cut-out seat and the slanting
back of the obstetric chair, which was formed so as to receive the patient in the same position which she was wont
to occupy on the lap of a fellow being.

We now come to the semi-recumbent position assumed
by the parturient woman whose labor takes places in the

obstetric chair, under the supervision of a midwife or phy-sician.

The obstetric chair marks a decided era in the history of the art ; but I must consider that period as a whole, and in speaking of the chair I have reference to its more charac-teristic features, to those points which are common to all ob-stetric chairs, as it is not my purpose here to describe the various obstetric chairs which were in use at different times,

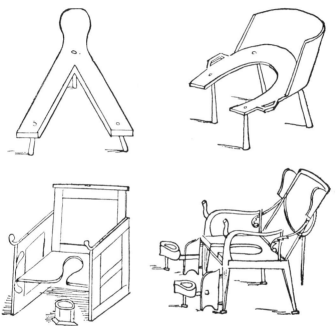

FIG. 31. — Development of the Obstetric Chair (from Goodell   Savonarola, 1547; Eucharius Rhodius, 1544; Deventer, 1701 ; Stein, 1805.

marking the progress of midwifery ; the modifications were too numerous. " As in our times," to use Dr. Goodell's very striking expression, " eminent physicians are seeking to improve the obstetric forceps, so in those days learned men did not disdain to perfect the *sella lochæa obstetricia seu obstetrica.*" My intention is merely to refer to the obstet-ric chair as being an artificial means of placing the patient in that semi-recumbent position which I deem most advantageous to the progress of labor, and which uncivilized people of the present day, as well as civilized nations of the past, long before the day of the chair, assumed as most comfortable for the parturient woman. The subject has been exhausted by the able pen of one of our fellows, Dr. Goodell, in his article on " Some Ancient Methods of Delivery;" and Dr. Ploss, in his work, gives so complete a history of this method of delivery that I need but refer briefly to the subject. The obstetric chair which flourished in the days of Greece and Rome was almost forgotten in the darkness of the earlier centuries of the Christian era, but seems to have survived in Italy, partly owing to the writing of Greek and Roman authorities, partly because the custom was handed down from generation to generation among the people ; and from Italy it found its way across the Alps into Germany and France. By this time, however, the rude stool of ancient times had been greatly changed in shape, complicated and improved, until the low stool, as we still see it in the hands of the Cypriote midwife, is presented to us as the typical obstetric chair of the Middle Ages.

The chair is mentioned by Albertus Magnus in the thirteenth century, and in the German translation of this work, under date of 1589, an illustration is given which resembles the obstetric chair of Soranus and Moschion. In the seventeenth and earlier part of the eighteenth century the chair seems to have flourished in Germany, and also in England, and numerous modifications were introduced. Its supremacy, however, was not of long duration, and it soon yielded to the modern recumbent position, and was only retained by the more conservative people in the rural districts, who follow but slowly in the wake of any advance. Smellie[1] says : " In remote parts of England the patient sat upon a stool made in the form of a semicircle." This, of course, was during the time of the decline of the chair, when the dorsal and lateral decubitus had become popular.

In the seventeenth century it was to be found in the centres of medical learning, and had not yet been forced back into the rural wilds.

[1] Vol. i., p. 203, 4th edition.

As a matter of curiosity, I will cite the title of a work published in 1637, in which it was warmly advocated, and I will add a brief description of the chair, in the quaint language of the book, kindly furnished me by Dr. Wise, of the Surgeon-general's Library, and it will answer for this as well as all other chairs, and will serve to show the importance attached to its various features.

"The Expert Midwife : or, an Excellent and most necessary Treatise of the Generation and Birth of Man. Wherein is contained many very Notable and Necessary Particulars requisite to be knowne and practiced : with Divers Apt and Useful Figures appropriated to this Worke. Also the Causes, signes, and Various Cures, of the most Principall Maladies and Infirmities incident to Women. Six Books compiled in Latine by the Industry of James Rueff, a Learned and Expert Chirurgion : and now translated into English for the Generall Good and Benefit of this Nation."

"Let the stoole be made compassewise, under-propped with foure feet, the stay of it behind bending backward, hollow in the midst, covered with a blacke cloth underneath, hanging downe to the ground, by that meanes that the labouring woman may be covered, and other women sometimes apply their hands in any place, if necessity require. Let the stoole be furnished and covered with many cloths and clouts at the back and other parts, that the labouring woman receive no hurt, or the infant anywhere, strongly kicking and striving because of the paines, stirrings and motions of the mother. And after the labouring woman shall be set in her chaire about to be delivered, the midwife shall place one woman behind her back which may gently hold the labouring woman, taking her by both the armes, and if need be, the pains waxing grievous, and the woman labouring, may stroke and presse downe the wombe, and may somewhat drive and depress the infant downward. But let her place other two by her sides, which may both, with good words, encourage and comfort the labouring woman, and also may be ready to helpe and put to their hand at any time. This being done, let the midwife herselfe sit stooping forward before the labouring woman, and let her annoint her own hands, and the womb of the labouring woman, with oile of lillies, of sweet almonds, and the grease of an hen, mingled and tempered together. For to doe this, doth profit and help them very much which are gross, and fat, and them whose secret parts are strict and narrow, and likewise them which have the mouth of the matrix dry, and such women as are in labour of their first child."

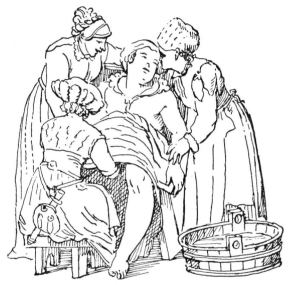

FIG. 32.—Delivery in the Obstetric Chair; after Rueffius. 1637.

The antiquity of the obstetric chair has been greatly overrated, owing to the misconception or misconstruction of the data in our possession. I have endeavored to give conscientiously the earliest positive references to the chair which we have, and that, I think, is by Moschion in the second century; but the votive group from the temple of Golgoi, in Cyprus (pictured and described above), and that famous passage from Exodus, both of which are quoted as evidences of the early use of the chair, will, I trust, cease to figure in that capacity.

The group from the Cesnola Collection has been fully

described in its proper place ; and as regards that oft-quoted passage from Exodus i. 15 and 16, which is referred to by so many writers as indicating the use of the obstetric chair among the ancient Hebrews ; it is translated by such, " When ye do the office of midwife to the Hebrew women, and see them upon the stool, if it be a son, then ye shall kill him," etc. I, however, believe, with Kotelman, that that word "*ebnaim,*" which is made so much of, and is'translated, as already stated, by many as *chair* or *stool,* means *stones.* So that the passage would read : " When ye see the woman upon the stones." This would prove, as is most probable, that it was the custom of the ancient Hebrews to be delivered, like the Arabs of the present day, as observed by Dr. Goguel and others, in the squatting posture, seated upon two stones. These details are more interesting than important, and it will certainly suffice, as far as the antiquity of the chair is involved, to state the fact that several Arab authorities recommended the obstetric chair in difficult labors, and that it was also advocated by Hippocrates and Soranus among the Greeks, who were usually confined in the semi-recumbent position, often in bed. These are the first authentic statements as to its use. Its history has been a checkered one. At the present day, the obstetric chair is popularly used only among the nations of the East, and, as Ploss says, " It is remarkable that it should be among the very people who rarely make use of a chair for sitting purposes." We find the chair now in use in Japan and China, in Turkey, Greece, Assyria, and Egypt. In Japan, it was still advocated by obstetricians in the last century ; in China it is common even now, although physicians battle against it. In Turkey it is used occasionally by certain midwives, as stated by P. Eram.[1] Dr. Denham speaks of its use in the East at the present day.[2] In Syria, no respectable midwife or "diyeh" is without her chair, as I am informed by Dr. A. J. A. Arbeely, of

[1] *Quelques considerations prat. sur les accouch. en Orient*, p. 407.

[2] Address before the Dublin Obstetric Society at its twenty-seventh annual session.

Damascus. The chair so used is different from any other
I have seen described, and appears to be a most practical
contrivance, enabling the woman to assume various inclinations of the body ; it is like a rocking-chair with comfortable arms, the seat about two feet above the rockers,
and cut out in a semicircle, so as to permit the expulsion of
the child. An assistant holds the parturient woman by sitting behind her, or at her side, whilst the midwife remains
in front to support the perineum with the palm of her hand,
greased with lard or olive oil.

I have already called attention to the fact that those na-

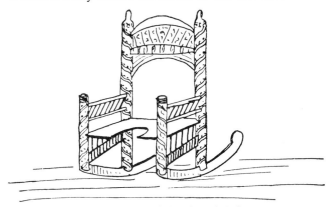

FIG. 33. — Obstetric Chair in use in Syria.

tions who resort to the chair in obstetric practice rarely
make use of it for ordinary purposes, and it appears highly
probable to me that the absence of the rocking-chair from
foreign homes may be accounted for by the fact that the
only rocking-chair of which they had cognizance was the
chair which the midwife carried from house to house, whenever her assistance was asked, for the relief of the child-
bearing woman ; this chair was then so intimately associated with the idea of suffering, of labor, and child-birth, that
it did not appear as a desirable piece of furniture for parlor
or sitting-room ; it would have seemed improper and out of
place. For similar reasons the comfortable arm-chair is an
unknown luxury among certain Eastern people.

It is only within late years that the American rocking-chair has found its way across the ocean, and the increased facilities for intercourse, and the spread of a leveling civilization, will soon do away with these remnants of former times which still linger here and there. Amongst the modern Egyptians, the midwife makes use of a chair, " Kursee El-Wiladeh," which is covered with a shawl, or an embroidered napkin, and some flowers of the henna tree, or some roses, are' tied with an embroidered handkerchief to each of the upper corners of the back; thus ornamented, the chair is conveyed before the midwife to the house. In the houses of the rich, the parturient is placed on a bed after delivery, and usually remains there from three to six days, whilst the poor women resume their ordinary occupation in a day or two.[1] I will add that Lane, like almost every other author, refers to that passage, Exodus i. 16, intending to compare the custom of using the chair among the Egyptians with that of the ancient Hebrews. In Palestine, the obstetric chair is still an honored institution, but much simplified in form, being sometimes nothing more than an old-fashioned arm-chair.

(*d.*) *Semi-recumbent Position, Strictly Speaking.*

Although I have grouped as semi-recumbent all the positions last spoken of, I will, in this subdivision, confine the use of the expression more closely, and will class as semi-recumbent, strictly speaking, only those positions in which the patient assumes the dorsal decubitus with the head and shoulders raised, the axis of the body inclined at an angle of about forty-five degrees.

Like many other of these curious positions, this one is found in our own States, but seems to have come to us from the French settlers in the north. In Vermont, some thirty years ago, a semi-recumbent position was customary, which may either be looked upon as a rude imitation of the obstetric chair, or as a semi-recumbent position, strictly

[1] E. W. Lane, *The Manners and Customs of the Modern Egyptians,* vol. ii., p. 306.

speaking, and probably the custom has not as yet entirely passed away ; the women in the rural districts were confined upon a bed made of three chairs tied together, upon which a straw bed was placed, and covered with a sheet. In front of this couch sat two women, whose duty it was to take the feet of the parturient woman in their laps, whilst the accoucheur sat between them, in front of the patient, where he was supposed to remain for two or three hours during the latter part of labor, if he did his whole duty.[1] The Canadian French women are partial to the in-

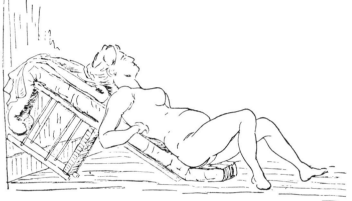

FIG. 34. — Favorite Posture of the French Canadian.

clined plane, made by turning forward and downward a high-backed chair, pressing it back against the wall of the room and making a bed upon it; though comfortable for the patient the legs of the attendant suffer from the stooping posture necessary.[2]

The custom in Japan, if I may judge from illustrations in a very complete " Japanese Midwifery," is a semi-recumbent position, on a mattress placed upon the floor, with the head and shoulders well elevated, so that the body is inclined at an angle of about forty or forty-five degrees. Precisely the same position is found among some of the Sioux nations,

[1] S. S. Clark, M. D., St. Albans, Vt.
[2] Dr. John Yale.

and the Assneboine Indians, who, as I am told by the well-known Indian interpreter, F. F. Gerard, lie on their backs, the head and shoulders propped at an angle of forty or forty-five degrees. This is the position usually assumed by them, although they are sometimes confined in the kneeling posture, like most Indians.

The Ute, Comanche, Apache, Navajoe, and Nez-Percés woman is also confined in the semi-recumbent dorsal position, the head and shoulders of the patient being frequently supported in the lap of an attendant, while the patient has access to a rope or brace placed within reach.[1]

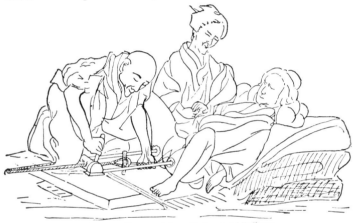

FIG. 35. — Japanese Labor. Instrumental Delivery.

Among the Pahutes, the parturient woman is placed in her tent, on blankets and skins, in a semi-reclining position, with her hips firm on the couch; she is supported by an assistant, who sits behind her, and in whose arms she reclines; her legs are flexed, and additional assistants hold and steady the knees; a leather girdle is fastened about her above the womb, and, as expulsive pains come on, three or more women push the girdle down after the escaping child.[2]

The Comanche woman gives birth to her child in some

1 Dr. L. Huntington, Surgeon U. S. A.
2 F. R. Waggoner, M. D.

secluded spot not far from the camp, in the dorsal decubitus, on a low extemporized couch prepared for her under a tree. Upon this she is placed, with her feet against the trunk of a tree, lying on her back. A lariat, a small rope of buffalo or raw hide, is thrown over a branch and secured; one end of it is placed in the hands of the woman, and she is allowed to pull through as best she may.[1] This would prove that during the pains, and the expulsion of the child, the patient raises herself by the lariat, and thus assumes the semi-recumbent position.

The Hindoos seem to find the position convenient, as the

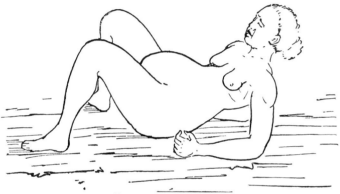

FIG. 36. — Penomonee Labor.

parturient woman is delivered while resting on her back, in the lap of a female seated on the ground, while her knees are bent, and are supported by two other females, one sitting on either side. In order to facilitate labor the parts are lubricated with oil, and the "Dyhe," resting on her knees before the patient, instead of supporting the perineum, urges the patient to assist nature in expelling the child, while she introduces the fingers of her two joined hands in a conical figure into the vagina, and, by spreading them, stretches the external parts, thinking in this way to facilitate labor, whilst she unquestionably retards it.[2] I

[1] H. S. Kilbourne, Assistant Surgeon U. S. A.

[2] "Notes on Hindoo Midwifery" by Dr. Wise, *Edinburgh Obstetrical Society, 12th Session,* p. 372.

will call especial attention to the custom of the Hoopa, lower Klamath, and the Orleans-Bar tribes, as it is precisely the same as I have occasionally seen my patients occupy in the efforts of expulsion. Lying on the back, the elbows drawn upwards and resting on the ground, the knees flexed to a perpendicular, the legs more or less flexed, and the heels resting on the ground.

The dorsal decubitus, with the body at an angle of forty or forty-five degrees, was common among the Romans. Moschion describes it. Celsius[1] and Paul of Ægina[2] recom-

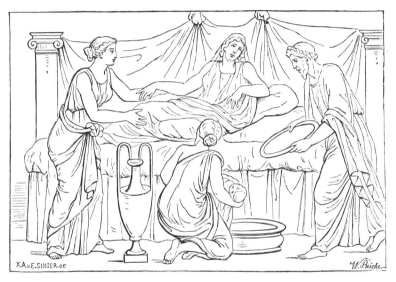

FIG. 37.— Birth of the Emperor Titus. From Ploss. After an antique painting on the ceiling of a room in the palace of Titus, on the Esquiline Hill in Rome.

mend this position in certain obstetrical operations, and before the time of the obstetric chair it was commonly assumed in Germany. In some of the mountainous districts of Saxony the patient, semi-recumbent, shoulders elevated, is suspended during the pains and the expulsion of the child, upon a strong broad towel which is placed under the pelvis and seems to further labor most happily in many

---

[1] Lib. 7, cap. xxix.   [2] Cap. vi., p. 74.

cases.[1] The Gurian women take the dorsal decubitus, but at the moment of expulsion seize a rope suspended above the bed and raise the body to the same angle which we have found among so many other people.[2] Most reasonable of all seems the semi-recumbent position as occasionally adopted in the rural districts of this country; the patient

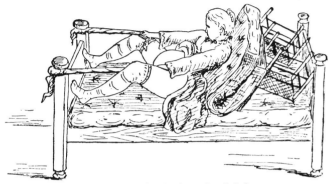

Fig. 38. — Virginia.   Semi-recumbent in bed.

being upon a bed doubled up against inverted chairs, the feet resting against the foot board, sheets or towels being fastened to the bed posts.

C. HORIZONTAL, OR RECUMBENT.

We finally come to the horizontal or recumbent position, and by this I mean especially, 1. *The Dorsal Decubitus*, the obstetric position of the present day on the continent of Europe and in America, the head merely elevated by the ordinary pillow ; 2. *The Position on the Side*, as customary in England; and 3. *Horizontal, Prone on the Chest and Stomach.*

1. *The Dorsal Decubitus.*

The semi-recumbent position held sway in Europe before the time of the obstetric chair, and after a period of great popularity soon disappeared, although its traces remained, especially in the slowly progressing country districts, until

[1] Dr. Leopold, *N. Ztschr. f. Geburtsk.*, xxv., 3, 1849.
[2] Ploss, 43.

the last thirty or forty years, when it finally yielded completely to the dorsal decubitus, which is now almost universal among civilized people. In England, where, however, it has now yielded almost entirely to the left lateral position, it began to grow in favor in the beginning of the last century ; in Scotland toward the end of that century. White, of Manchester, it may be of interest to note, was the first to advocate the dorsal and lateral decubitus in England (1773).

The Chinese women are frequently confined in bed.[1]

Although this is the position which is taught by the laws of modern obstetrics, so perfect in all other respects, nature does not seem to have designed that woman should in this way free herself from her burden ; at least it appears very strange that instinct, the correct guide of uncivilized people, should so rarely lead them to adopt the recumbent position ; and it appears strange that, notwithstanding the most careful inquiry as to the position adopted by the savages, and notwithstanding the information I have received from surgeons who have come in contact with all of our Indian tribes, I have found scarcely any who assume a strictly recumbent position. Among some the women are confined in the dorsal decubitus, but rarely in the horizontal position. Among the Cheyennes and Arapahoes we sometimes find the dorsal decubitus in simple labors.[2] The Oregon Indians on the Siletz Reservation are invariably confined on the back with the feet drawn up. I am also told that others of the tribes on the Pacific coast follow this custom, especially those of the Grand Ronde Agency, Oregon ; the parturient usually keeps on her feet during the first stage of labor, but when the expulsion pains set in she lies on her back, her head very slightly elevated (her bed always on the floor), her thighs well flexed on the abdomen ; an assistant supports each knee and foot ; the patient presses her hands against her thighs, or, when the pains become severe, she presses

[1] Dabry, *La Médicine chez les Chinois*, Paris, 1863, p. 354.
[2] J. H. Bannister, M. D.

upon the fundus uteri ; later an assistant carefully manipu-, lates the fundus and follows the uterine globe.[1]

The Nez-Percés and Gros-Ventre squaw assumes the stooping posture during the earlier stages of labor, with an assistant at her back, who clasps her body with her arms, and locking the fingers, brings the palms of the hands over the base, of the uterus, making steady pressure backwards and downwards during the pains ; in some instances, during the stage of expulsion, however, the patient lies down indifferently on either side or on the back, while if on the side, pressure by the hands of the assistant is kept up continuously, if on the back, the assistant remains by the side of the patient and. keeps up the pressure in the before-mentioned directions.

Upon the Antilles the recumbent position is also assumed, though we have seen that other postures are equally common there. Among one of the African tribes, the Wanika, the parturient woman lies flat upon her back, and this is perhaps the only instance where the horizontal position is so decidedly described.[2] Of the Indian women, Susruta says, page 368, " When the child is to be born, let the woman be placed with the back upon a carefully spread couch, giving her a pillow, let the thighs be flexed, and let her be delivered by four steady, aged, and knowing midwives whose nails are well trimmed."

In Southern India we find a similar custom to that observed among the Nez-Percés ; the patient walks about in the earlier stages, then sits down with the legs stretched, her back supported by an assistant, whilst in the moment of expulsion she is placed upon her back.[3]

In Siam the patient is placed upon her back with a woman seated upon either side ; these two assistants begin by forcibly pressing the abdomen downward and backward, the pressing of which is continued from three to five hours. If by that time it has failed to expel the fetus, one attend-

[1] Dr. J. Fields.
[2] Hildebrandt.
[3] Shortt, *Edinb. M. J.*, Dec., 1862, p. 554.

ant is supported by the hand while she tramps the abdomen of the patient, always placing her feet above the fetus, as a *dernier ressort.* All other means having failed, they suspend the parturient by means of a band beneath the arms, as we have already mentioned.[1]

The Burmese practice is to strip the patient naked and to compel her to run about the room, while half a dozen

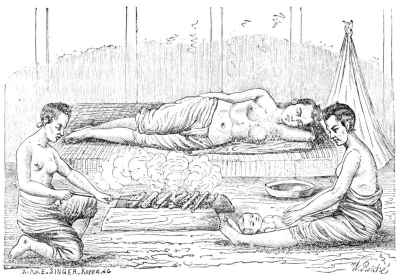

FIG. 39.—Couch and Lying-in Chamber of the Siamese. From Ploss.

women are about who squeeze her abdomen and beat it with pillows; this process is continued until finally she falls upon the floor exhausted, and some of the women still keep pressing the child down with their hands, trying to expel it forcibly; and there are instances, as the author is credibly informed, in which the woman is placed upon her back and the midwife sits upon her or stands up and presses against the child with one of her feet.[2]

In Australia other positions are assumed in simple labor,

[1] "Siamese Obstetrics," by W. L. Huntington, of Bangcock, Siam. *Med. Rec.,* N. Y., 1876, p. 133.
[2] *India J. M. Sc.,* Jan 1, 1835, p. 339.

but it seems that in difficult cases the parturient woman is treated in the same barbarous way. She lies upon her back between two assistants, one of whom places her knee in the small of the patient's back, whilst the other, lying more in front, awaits a labor pain and then presses her knees into the patient's abdomen.[1]

In Astrakhan the Russian women are made to walk about unceasingly during the earlier stages, and only at the very last moment are permitted to lie down.

In Sumatra, if we may judge from a single case,[2] the patient is also confined in the recumbent position ; and in Brazil, according to an old authority cited by Ploss,[3] the native women were confined upon the ground. Several other such vague authorities are cited, but they are hardly sufficiently reliable for our purpose.

2. *The Lateral Decubitus.*

The position upon the side seems almost entirely a product of modern civilization, and, I must say, of prudery rather than science; it is not adopted as the obstetric position by any of those people who still lead a natural life, though assumed, in a few rare instances, in certain stages of labor. The Nez-Percés squaws squat in the earlier stages, and lie upon the side or back during the expulsion of the child. The Modocs, on the contrary, first lie upon the side, and at the last moment take the knee-hand position. The women of the Laguna Pueblo, New Mexico, who follow their own inclination almost altogether in the position which they assume, stand or walk about in the early stages, but are confined standing, suspended in a half squatting position, or, if tired, on the back or side, with pillows between the knees ; this latter position is also occasionally found among the Kootenai Indians, of Washington Territory ; as Dr. Morgan writes, the woman is placed on her left side, under

---

[1] Marston, *Journal of the Ethnological Society*, London, 1869–70. Ploss, p. 14.

[2] *Monatschr. f. Geburtsk. u. Frauenkr.*, viii., p. 3.

[3] Jean de Laet, 1640.

which is placed a pillow, or bundle of skins; another roll of skins, or a blanket, is between her knees, which are separated, so as to be about a foot apart; the patient holds a stake or cord, the arms are flexed, and the head touches the hands.

With the exception of these few data, I can find no other reference to this position.

3. *Prone upon the Stomach.*

This peculiar position has but few adherents; in fact, I can find no traces of it elsewhere than among the Creeks, who assume an over-done knee-chest position; *i. e.*, prone upon chest and stomach, in ordinary cases. "When the fetus is about to be expelled the mother straps the belt

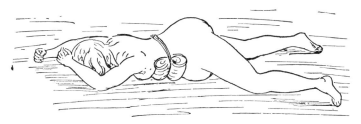

Fig. 40. — Crow-Creek. Prone upon face and abdomen, across a pillow.

across her chest, allowing it to extend somewhat on to the abdomen. As the labor proceeds the strap is buckled tighter and tighter, until the expulsion is accomplished; meantime the position assumed by the mother is prone upon her face, her chest and abdomen across the pillow; in this position she remains until the expulsion. She then stands up, resting on a stick of some sort, with the feet spread wide apart. This is to let the blood flow more freely, and, so they think, to allow the placenta to be more rapidly and easily delivered." [1]

Upon the Island of Ceram, as well as in Loango, and other districts of Central Africa, the patient is placed upon her stomach if labor does not progress in the ordinary posi-

[1] Dr. M. P. Pomeroy, Crow-Creek Agency, D. T.

tion, and the expulsion. of the child is hastened by kneading or tramping upon the back of the sufferer.

A peculiar custom may yet be mentioned which is still observed, to the great discomfort of the parturient woman, among some of our western Indians, as well as among the more civilized natives of Syria ; and that is, to toss the suffering patient in a blanket, the four corners of which are held by stout men, so that she is well shaken, with a view, probably, of rectifying the malposition, and shaking out the fetus from the unwilling womb.

PART II.

The Position of Women among Civilized Races of the Present Day in the Agony of the Expulsive Pains.

Abler obstetricians than myself have undoubtedly understood the movements of women, and the positions which they assumed in the agony of the expulsive pains. As regards myself, I must candidly confess this was not the case ; and it was not until I had undertaken this work, and had begun to study the positions assumed by savage and civilized people during labor, that I began to understand that there was a method in the instinctive movements of women in the last stage of labor. I had seen them toss about, and sought to quiet them ; I bade them have patience, and lie still upon their backs ; but, since entering upon this study, I have learned to look upon their movements in a very different light. I have watched them with interest and profit, and believe that I have learned to understand them. It has often appeared to me, as I sat watching a tedious labor case, how unnatural was the ordinary obstetric position for the parturient woman ; the child is forced, I may say, upwards through the pelvic canal in the face of gravity, which acts in the intervals between the pains, and permits the presenting part of the child to sink back again, down the inclined canal. If we look upon the structure of the pelvis, more especially the direction of the pelvic canal and its axis, if we take into consideration the assistance which may be rendered by gravity, and, above all, by the abdominal muscles, the present obstetric position seems indeed a peculiar one.

The contractions of the previously inactive and rested abdominal muscles are a powerful adjunct to the tired uterine fibre, in the last prolonged and decisive expulsory effort, and in the dorsal decubitus they are somewhat hampered ; they act to the best advantage in the inclined positions, semi-recumbent, kneeling, or squatting. We know that the squatting position is the one naturally assumed if an effort is required to expel the contents of the pelvic viscera ; we, moreover, all know how difficult, even impossible, it is for many to perform those functions recumbent in bed, and mainly because they have not sufficient control of the abdominal muscles in that position. Much more is this the case in the expulsion of the child ; but the recumbent position is sanctioned by custom ; it is pointed out as apparently convenient; it is imperatively demanded by prudery, and by a false modesty which hides from view the patient's body beneath the bed-clothes ; and above all it is dictated by modern laws of obstetrics, the justice of which I have never dared question; we have all been taught their correctness, and we all thoughtlessly follow their dictates. There is no reason for assuming this position, though we are taught it ; it is not reason, or obstetric science, but obstetric fashion which guides us, — guides us through our patients ; and blindly do we, like all fashion's votaries, follow in the wake.

We have seen in the first part of this paper that the recumbent position is one but rarely taken by women among savage tribes, or among people who still follow their instinct and not the dictates of the latest obstetric fashion. Now what does civilized woman in the hands of the modern obstetrician do when in the intense agony of the last expulsive pains ? She loses control of herself, forgets the admonition of her physician, and gives way to her own in-

stinct. You have all seen what I have learned to understand but recently. The parturient woman, at the time of
the expulsive pains, raises herself in bed into a semi-recumbent position upon her hands or elbows. This struck me
most forcibly when I observed this motion in a young primipara who had gone through the earlier stages of labor
bravely, and although partially under the influence of chlo-
roform, when, with the last severe pains the head of the
child would advance and then again recede, she finally, in

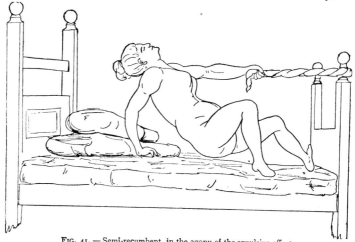

FIG. 41. — Semi-recumbent, in the agony of the expulsive effort

her agony raised herself up into a semi-recumbent position,
resting on her arms, and with the next pain the child was
born.

Other women assume this semi-recumbent position by
clinging to the neck of the husband, or an assistant who
may be seated by the bedside. It is not love for the person which dictates this motion ; it is an instinctive desire
to raise herself into a semi-recumbent position, to facilitate
the expulsion of the burden she bears. Others, again, have
a sheet or rope fastened to the bedpost, upon which they
pull with their arms ; the object of this is only to assist in
the effort of raising herself partially in bed, into a semi-recumbent position, as the kneeling savage raises herself by

a rope which is fastened above her head, or as others recumbent in bed or upon the floor, half raise themselves
by a rope or pole above the head. It was instinct, certainly not obstetric teaching, which told the patients referred to by Dr. Campbell to assume the squatting position
by which they were so easily delivered of their children,
whilst tedious labor stared them in the face if they obeyed
the modern obstetric fashion. In one case it was a negro,
in the other it was a white woman of high social standing,
who had suffered in several tedious labors while obliged to
follow the dictates of her physician to remain in her bed ;
in her agony, following her instinct, regardless of advice or
appearances, she assumed the squatting position, and was
easily delivered. In another case Dr. Campbell refers to a
girl whom he had lately confined kneeling upon the floor,
her arms resting upon a low rocking-chair. Being asked
how she came to assume this position, she said that in a
former labor, four years ago, the midwife had kept her
strictly in bed, never allowing her to get up ; this, however,
she was able to do occasionally, when the pains always
seemed to improve. She said that the midwife threatened
to tie her in bed if she did not remain quiet. She was, upon
that occasion, in labor from four o'clock in the afternoon
until ten o'clock of the second day ; being in great distress,
she disobeyed the midwife, and left her bed ; her pains immediately increased, and she knelt down on the floor with
her face resting in the lap of her mistress, and was in the
same position as with the chair in the following labor ; she
says that she had not been in that position more than five
minutes before the child was born. Her expression was,
" The floor is the best place to have a baby, and I don't
think I ever could have one in bed." The woman seemed
quite intelligent, and afterwards candidly stated that her
first thought, on the doctor's entering the room, was a dread
that she would be put to bed and stopped from completing
her labor.

I need hardly continue this evidence, as every one of the
members is aware how frequently, in the last moments, a

change of position is made by the agonized woman. Rarely the inclined position, kneeling, or squatting, is assumed, mostly the semi-recumbent position, and that is the one which seems dictated by the instinct of the patient, and the one which I would accordingly advocate.

RÉSUMÉ AND CONCLUSIONS.

I WILL briefly recall the more striking and important features elicited in the inquiries I have made in regard to the posture of women in labor.

I. *The women of the various tribes and races are delivered according to customs, and in positions, which are peculiar to their people, whenever they are free to follow their own instincts.*

(*a*.) These positions are now adopted as customary and traditional, but in the first place they were assumed because they had proved the safest and best ; delivery, in simple cases, being thus accomplished in the shortest possible time with the least possible suffering.

(*b*.) So great do the advantages of posture in childbirth seem to be, that people cling to this custom more firmly than to any other of their traditions, as we have seen by the chair of the Cypriote midwife, who to-day reënacts the labor scene of 2,300 years ago ; and of the native Peruvian woman, who is still confined as were her ancestors at the time of the Incas.

II. *The positions assumed in civilized communities, by the advice of learned authorities, have varied greatly with the change in obstetric science, and with the demands of comfort and of modesty ;* thus, in the days of Greece and Rome, in the early centuries of the Christian era, a semi-recumbent position was advocated, either upon a low stool or in bed ; later came the obstetric chair, and toward the end of the last century the dorsal decubitus, which has retained its supremacy, yielding, however, to the position on the side in the British Isles, and to the dictates of Nature in the agonies of the expulsive pains, when women will occasionally disobey the conscientious obstetrician, that they may obtain speedy relief.

III. *The same woman often assumes various position in the course of a natural labor ; usually, she is more at her ease in the early stages, and not until the pains become more regular, rapid, and severe, does she take the position in which she is confined.*

Thus, the Coyotero-Apache squaw occupies any position she pleases, generally standing or walking about until bearing-down pains supervene (which, in fact, is almost universal among the North American Indians), then she assumes the squatting posture. The squaws of the Laguno Pueblo stand with their hands on their knees, much as they urinate, in the earlier stages ; later, they stand up erect, supported by assistants or clinging to a rope. The Modocs maintain a curved position, lying on the side, until the labor is nearly completed, when they assume a position on their knees and hands, which is continued until the child is born.

Among the Nez-Percés and Gros-Ventres the parturient is in a stooping posture during the first two stages of labor, the buttocks resting on the heels, whilst during the expulsion of the child she lies down, on either side, or on the back.

IV. *In the last stages of ordinary labor, those positions which I have classified as inclined are most frequently resorted to ;* most common of all is the kneeling position, which we mainly find among the Tartars, Mongolians, and North American Indians : the squatting posture is also at home among our Indians, and among the Malays, the Australian and African negroes ; equally frequent are the semi-recumbent positions, which, although resorted to by savage nations, are more closely connected with the progress of civilization. The ruder methods, such as the semi-recumbent position in the lap of an assistant, or on the ground, answer the same purpose as the more comfortable and refined posture in the obstetric chair or in bed.

Least frequent are the recumbent or horizontal, and the standing or erect postures.

V. *In all positions, whether the patient is swinging by the limb of a tree, whether she is kneeling by a stake, or semi-recumbent in bed, there is a decided change in the axis of the body during the pain, and in the interval of rest; and usually the patient has a support of some kind within reach, a rope, a stake, or an assistant, by means of which she can change the axis of the body, and intensify the contractions of voluntary and involuntary muscles during the pains.*

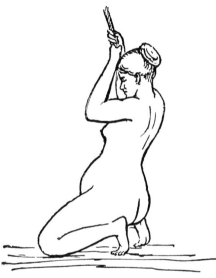

FIG. 42. — Kneeling, clinging to rope.

The pelvis itself is usually steadied, whilst the upper portion of the trunk sways to and fro.

Some of our Indians walk about in the interval, and kneel down, clinging to the stake during the pain; for this purpose the Comanches, for instance, have a number of stakes planted in the ground at the place of confinement, in order that the patient may walk about, and still find a support to kneel by at any moment, when the pain overtakes her.

The weakly woman, among the Kootenai Indians, who is confined in a recumbent position, raises herself by a rope which is suspended above her during the severer pains, and during the expulsion of the child.

The Indians on the Mexican frontier, who are confined in a kneeling position, usually stand or recline on the bed during the interval between the pains; but when a pain is coming on, they immediately grasp the convenient rope and hang on with all their might; and this position permits of the easiest and freest motion of the body for the purpose of best adapting the inclination of the pelvic axis to demands of the advancing head.

The native Mexican is often confined kneeling on the floor ; in the interval between the pains she lets herself down, her buttocks resting upon her heels, whilst during the pain she raises the body, throwing it backward or forward, according to circumstances, and clings to a rope, an assistant, or the neck of the midwife.

Surgeon George W. Adair, U. S. A., justly characterizes the difference in the methods pursued by various people. He says : " The English midwife exhorts the patient to lean forward; in America, the feet are fixed, and the patient is given a rope by which she raises herself during the pain ; the Mexican midwife fixes the knees and holds the upper portion of the trunk as in a vice, and pulls the pelvis forward, hinged, as it were, upon the acetabulum, and thus overcomes the dip of the plane of the superior strait, and straightens the passage with greater efficiency and certainty."

Dr. Campbell closely observed the negro woman whom he saw confined in a kneeling posture, her arms resting upon a low chair, and saw that during the pain her body would move backwards so that her buttocks would rest between her heels, while in the intervals she would glide forward again, so that the thighs became perpendicular and the body horizontal.

VI. *In tedious cases, when delivery is retarded and labor will not advance, a change is usually made in the posture of the patient, and massage is freely resorted to ;* thus, the Cheyennes, Arapahoes, Nez-Percés, and Gros Ventres, who assume the dorsal decubitus in ordinary labor cases, raising themselves into a semi-recumbent position during the expulsion of the child, resort to the knee-elbow position in difficult cases.

The Siamese, who usually assume the recumbent position, and our Coyotero-Apaches, who squat in ordinary cases, both suspend the parturient by bands about the chest, if labor is delayed, and let several assistants cling to the sufferer, suspending themselves from her with their arms above the uterine tumor ; the Siamese draw their patient up in an erect posture, whilst the Apache squaw is swung in a more kneeling position.

Upon the Pacific slope, where the dorsal decubitus is the rule in ordinary cases, the patient is partially suspended in a kneeling or squatting position in difficult cases ; the Syrians, who usually permit their patients the comforts of the obstetric rocking-chair, toss them in a blanket to shake the child out, or turn it, if the labor becomes tedious.

Instinct and experience teach the savage that by a change of position, labor may be hastened or retarded, and involuntarily they change the axis of the body in a way most favorable to a natural and safe delivery, hastening labor as much as is compatible with the safety of mother and child ; all the inclined positions, especially the kneeling and squatting, clinging to a rope, are such that the direction of the pelvic axis can be readily changed. It remains for the scientific observer to demonstrate with precision the positions which are the most favorable under given conditions.

Herr von Ludwig, the speculative and theoretical writer, who has been condemned and ignored by practical obstetricians, describes the knee-elbow position as the one which retards the expulsion, making it slower and safer in difficult cases, saving the perineum, and the kneeling position, with the body inclined forward, as the one which retards expulsion but moderately, with proper care of the perineum.

Although it is not within the scope of this study to discuss the question as to the best position for women in labor, we may well look to the ethnological facts cited for a solution of this puzzling and highly important problem, and I will outline the more important *conclusions* which have developed.

I. *In the ordinary labor case, which is a purely mechanical process, the patient should be given greater liberty and should be permitted to follow the dictates of her instinct*

in regard to her movements more freely than is now cus-
tomary.

II. *In the earlier stages of labor the parturient must be*
guided in her actions, and in the position assumed, by her
own comfort and by the dictates of her instinct ; not only is
this the invariable rule among savage races, but it was also
warmly advocated by the shrewd and observing obstetricians of the past, and by those eminently practical and successful midwives of old.

III. *The care with which the parturient women of unciv-*
ilized people avoid the dorsal decubitus, the modern obstetric
position, at the termination of labor, is sufficient evidence that
it is a most undesirable position for ordinary cases of confine-
ment ; and I am convinced that the thinking obstetrician will
soon confirm the statement not unfrequently made by the
ignorant but observing savage, by Negro and Indian, that the
recumbent position retards labor and is inimical to easy, safe,
and rapid delivery.

Several of the most esteemed of my colleagues have already given me a very decided expression of their opinion,
taking the same grounds practically and theoretically. Dr.
Campbell, of Georgia, says that a careful study of the actions of parturient woman in her natural state will force
us to permit our patients, sometimes, at least, to obey their
own impulses, and to assume a squatting, kneeling, or sitting posture, in their attempts to deliver themselves ; and
this, he adds, "would, in my opinion, often do away with the
necessity of resorting to the forceps, which, though a great
blessing, too often become the reverse in the hands of eager
obstetricians, who are inclined to use them on the least occasion, or without any real occasion at all." He has given
me the history of a number of cases, most of which I have
already cited, in which labor was retarded, progress had entirely ceased, and the propriety of the forceps was under
consideration, when a speedy and unaided delivery followed
a change of position from the routine dorsal decubitus to
the squatting, sitting, or kneeling posture, as the instinct of
the patient prompted ; but be it remembered, the same pa-

tient, when free to follow her instinct, always adopted the same position.

The cases related by Dr. Campbell are as striking as the one told me by Dr. V. Mansfelde, of Kansas : the patient being in great distress, labor having continued for several days, entire cessation of pains in the usual obstetric position, their sudden recurrence upon assumption of an inclined position, their disappearance, with the certainty of a chemical experiment, upon a return to the dorsal decubitus, and final speedy delivery in the position of the patient's choice.

Dr. Wilcox, of Massachusetts, and others have related similar cases, most of which I have already given, but I cannot close without again referring to the views of my friend, Dr. Campbell : " I will say that I regard what may be called the *Obstetric position*, as generally practised in this country, recumbent on the back, as not only the most unnatural, but the most disadvantageous and therefore the most unphilosophical ; it is the position which, above all others, deprives the woman in labor of the advantages which gravity would give us in promoting expulsion ; there the position almost nullifies the power of the abdominal muscles, leaving the almost unassisted uterine muscle to effect expulsion. The English method, on the side with the body bent forward and the thighs drawn up, is much more advantageous in so far as the abdominal muscles can act better."

IV. *In ordinary labor cases the expulsion of the child should be expected in an inclined position: Kneeling, squatting or semi-recumbent, in bed, on the chair or lap, as is done by the great majority of uncivilized people, and for the following reasons : —*

a. These positions permit the free use of the abdominal muscles.

b. The force of gravity does not counteract the expulsive effort as in the recumbent position, nor does it unite with it too freely, and hasten labor unduly, as in the erect posture.

c. With the assistance of a rope, stake, or other support the parturient can vary the inclination of the body and correct the labor, hasten or retard the descent of the child, and relieve the pain, changing the axis of the body and throwing the fetal head toward the sacrum or symphysis.

d. Injury to the soft parts is less liable to occur in these positions, if we may accept the rapid getting up, and freedom of our Indian squaw from all uterine diseases, as proof of this statement.

V. *Of these positions the semi-recumbent is the most serviceable, and should be adopted as the obstetric position in all ordinary labor cases ; it is preferable to the kneeling or squatting.*

a. As more convenient and comfortable, not exposing the person, and not being objectionable to the modesty of the patient.

b. As affording more rest and not being tiresome, which is a serious objection to the kneeling and squatting position as applicable to the tender female of our civilization.

c. The semi-recumbent position in bed, the body at an angle of forty-five degrees, the hips resting on a hard mattress, thighs well flexed, is the easiest, most comfortable, and appears to afford the greatest relief, and the greatest freedom from pain, coupled with the greatest effect of the uterine contractions, relaxation of all the parts, and free play of the abdominal muscles.

d. The pelvis is more readily fixed in this position.

e. The perineum has a certain support which does away with the questionable proceeding of supporting the perineum during expulsion of the head and shoulders, by which more harm than good is usually done.

THE

THIRD STAGE OF LABOR.

LABOR seems completed with the expulsion of the child, the one act upon which the efforts of the accoucheur and the expectations of the patient have centred, the culmination of hours of suffering and anxiety ; both feel as if their work were completed, and but little thought is given by either to the remaining afterbirth which is usually expelled without much suffering to the mother, and if nature be not interfered with, rarely calls for any exertion on the part of the attendant.

Accidents occurring during the birth of the child are immediately followed by alarming results, while those happening during the delivery of the placenta can be ignored at the time, although the consequences are often disastrous. The third stage of labor accordingly excites but little interest, and is, I may almost say, unduly neglected ; some radical changes have of late years been made in its treatment, but, although advocated by able obstetricians, they have by no means met with the hearty concurrence of the profession at large, of which they deserve and which their importance justifies.

My attention has been recently directed to what I may call the natural management of labor, or the customs observed during childbirth by such people as are not yet governed by modern obstetric law, and who follow the dictates of instinct in this purely mechanical function of our animal existence ; my researches in regard to the position of women in labor have shown me the correctness of the course adopted by those untutored people with whom methods have been traditionary for ages which have not until now reached us, in this advanced nineteenth century, as the teachings of our most scientific obstetricians; and I deem it of interest, if not of some little practical importance, to study the management of the placenta, indeed the treatment of the patient during the third stage of labor, among uncivilized people who are as yet forced to rely upon their instinct for their obstetric practice, and upon whom the obstetric laws, and I may-say obstetric fashions, of to-day have not yet encroached. It is only of late that ethnological studies have developed and have brought to light the innermost life and most private and secret customs of those interesting children of nature; but very little attention has, however, been paid to their obstetric practices, and above all to this very uninteresting and unimportant detail.

The management of the third stage of labor has received so little attention that I shall be obliged to confine myself, by reason of the scanty data at my command, to the leading points; I nevertheless hope to be able to develop the more important features sufficiently to show that these untutored people, following the guidance of instinct, have, as a rule, pursued a much more correct practice than can be attributed to the followers of scientific midwifery; above all they have fully appreciated, in resorting to abdominal expression, the dangers of the *vis a fronte*, and the importance of the *vis a tergo* as their main reliance for the speedy and su·cessful removal of the placenta. Nor are the data as broad as I should like to see them; I can gather but little from the records of travellers or from the pages of history; the information I have been able to obtain is almost altogether in regard to the customs now observed among the North American Indians, and for this I am indebted to the kindly interest shown by the surgeons of the United States Army, and the physicians of the Indian Agencies who have freely responded to the questions I have put in the circular sent out through the Smithsonian Institution by the generous offices of Major J. W. Powell, the director, and others of the gentlemen connected with the Bureau of Ethnology, above all Dr. H. C. Yarrow.

I shall discuss, first, the management of the third stage of labor in simple cases, as it is customary among the various tribes, and this will be best understood by describing, I., those methods which are adopted for the purpose of expelling the placenta, in which the patient retains the same position which she occupied in the delivery of the child, and, of these, the one ordinarily practised is by the employment of a *vis a tergo*, most commonly by a force applied externally from above downwards, by manual expression ; and secondly, by action of the diaphragm, by the use of emetics. Much less frequent is the employment of the *vis a fronte*, that fatal traction upon the cord, which forms the third group. Somewhat different from these methods is a fourth, which I have classified under II., comprising the customs of all those tribes who look upon a change of posture as the important element for the purpose of accomplishing the expulsion of the after-birth ; a change of position is made immediately after the birth of the child, and the patient assumes a different posture from the one occupied during the earlier stages of labor. This is not frequent in ordinary cases, but is a usual resort in case that some difficulty is experienced in the removal of the placenta. I have then considered under different heads the treatment of simple and difficult cases, and will next review the management of the cord, as it may be of interest to note the usual time of cutting the cord and the methods of cutting and tying it ; finally I will briefly indicate some of the more peculiar customs, and the, to us, strange views entertained with regard to this stage of labor.

MANAGEMENT OF SIMPLE CASES.

The placenta delivered in the same position which has been occupied during labor pains and the expulsion of the child.

Manual expression.—Among our Indians, as among all uncivilized nations, external manipulations are resorted to wherever good can be accomplished by them, and in obstetric practice massage and expression are freely and effectively used. The third stage of labor is a very short one, the placenta usually escaping very soon after the birth of the child ; and by far the most common, the prevailing treatment in fact, is the one we will now consider. The patient and her assistants retain the positions relatively occupied during the birth of the child ; the parturient, as is commonly the case, kneeling, whilst an assistant, who kneels or stands behind her, with her arms around her waist and the palms of her hands upon the fundus of the uterus, keeps up a steady pressure upon the contracting organ, and in case that the muscular action is not sufficient for the expulsion of the after-birth, she hastens its progress by an effective kneading. Moreover, we know that the kneeling, squatting, and semi-recumbent positions are those in which the abdominal muscles can be most effectively used for the purpose of expelling any of the contents of the abdominal cavity. This is true of the Commanches, of the Klamath, the Crows, Nez-Percés, Peorias, Shawnees, of the Kiowa, Caddo, Delaware, Wyandotte, Ottawa and Seneca tribes. The Clatsops carry out this idea perhaps even more effectively by placing a bandage about the patient's abdomen immediately after the expulsion of the child, " to keep the placenta from going back further into the body." And I may here state that this is the ruling idea in their treatment, as they dread such an accident very much, and unless the placenta is speedily delivered, the uterus responding to their manipulations, they are at a loss what more to do, and the patient is usually left to her fate, rarely escaping the consequent septicemia. The Dakotas permit the patient, if exhausted by the labor, to leave the kneeling posture and lie down during this last stage. Some of the tribes belonging to the great Sioux nation—the Blackfeet, Uncpapas, and the lower aud upper Yanktonans—follow this most judicious mode of delivering the afterbirth. In case that steady pressure from above downwards upon the fundus, and kneading of the tumor, does not suffice, the abdomen is rudely kneaded with the clenched fists, in various directions, in their endeavor to push the placenta out, as I gather from an interesting description of a case of retarded delivery of the placenta among the Umpynas.

The Kootewais kneel during labor, and after expulsion of the child continue to knead the abdomen, exercising the same pressure downward as when aiding the descent of the child, and in case this fails, they introduce the hand into the vagina and remove the placenta, giving the woman one joint of an unknown root to stop the hemorrhage, following it by another joint in fifteen minutes or half an hour until it does stop, with the idea

of checking the hemorrhage gradually. They let the patient
bleed to a certain extent, and if it exceeds their idea of what
she may well lose, they give the root. No reason is given
why they should not stop the bleeding at once. This is one
of the very few tribes who have any knowledge of the removal of the placenta by the introduction of the hand in
utero. The Papagos also seem to remove the placenta forcibly, if it does not speedily come by natural means. The
squaws of several tribes are delivered in a squatting posture,
and among them, also, the placenta is delivered precisely as
the child was, the patient and her assistants retaining the
same position, and the same pressure and manipulations being
kept up. This is true of the women of the Laguna-Pueblo,
of the Coyotero-Apaches, and some of the tribes of the
Sioux nation. The Brulé, Loafer, Agallala, Wazahzah, and
Northern—among these, as well as other of the Sioux tribes,
and the Kiowas, also, a change of posture is made. The
squaw belt is often used, and the placenta is delivered almost
immediately after the child, by the gradual tightening of the
broad leather belt, which is strapped above the womb as soon
as the child has appeared.

The women of the lower order of Mexicans, who are also
usually delivered in the squatting posture, sometimes kneeling,
follow the same custom as their Indian neighbors, but of
them I am told that the third stage of labor is a much longer
one. 'The midwife busies herself about the new-born child,
while the patient is kept in her uncomfortable position, kneeling or squatting, with her rear and lateral assistants, until the
placenta is expelled. This takes place seldom in less than half
an hour, but generally within an hour; if not, the patient receives a more or less violent shaking, according to the exigencies of the case, the rear assistant, with her arms about the
patient, actually shaking her up and down, and, if this does
not answer, as a last resort, efforts are made to provoke vomiting. A decoction of some kind, either laxative or nauseat-
ing, is given the patient for the purpose of assisting the expulsion of the placenta ; but among the Mexicans a cup of corn
gruel, *atole*, is regularly given after the expulsion of the child.
Among those who retain the semi-recumbent position in which
they are usually delivered are the Wacos, Hoopas, lower

Klamath, and Penimonce. This is a convenience for the midwife or assistant, as she can also assume a more comfortable position, and knead the abdomen to better purpose.

The Indians of the Pacific coast follow the same custom, and they, as well as all other tribes, seem anxious to attempt the speedy expulsion of the placenta, so that an effort is always made to assist the uterus in casting off the remaining afterbirth as soon as the child has been removed, and placed in a safe place. The accoucheur makes gentle, but tolerably firm traction on the cord with one hand, and with the other manipulates the abdomen over the uterine globe. At the same time, if thought necessary, the assistant will gently press the abdomen; both hands, with the distended fingers, being laid above

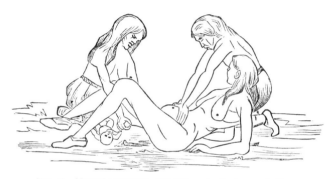

Fig. 43.—Manual expression of the placenta, Penimonee Indians.

the womb. At times, he does still more by kneading, with a view to pressing the secundines out of the uterine cavity, but if these efforts fail while the patient is in their usual obstetric position, the semi-recumbent, she is raised to an erect position, and then, well supported, the manipulations of the uterine globe are continued, and a more firm traction is made upon the cord.

Of the Flat-heads and Pend-oreilles, I am told that the placenta, in almost every case, is delivered with neither massage nor expression nor traction on the cord, nature, unaided completing the labor; very decided means are, however resorted to in case delay should occur, which is very rare Among those who assume the semi-recumbent position are also the Utes, Navajoes, Apaches, and some of the Nez-Percés, who assist nature by kneading the abdomen, but rarely by actual expression or traction upon the cord; they, however, expect to hasten the expulsion by anointing the abdomen with greasy unguents or decoctions of herbs.

The Burmese are among the very few people who adopt a *dorsal decubitus* as the obstetric position, and forcibly expel the placenta more by beating the abdomen than well-directed manipulations, and in extreme cases, by sitting or standing upon the abdomen and pressing with the feet upon the uterine globe.

The Makahs, of the Neah-Bay agency, retain the sitting posture in which the child is delivered, but whilst this, to them, apparently simple proceeding is always managed without professional assistance of any kind, skilled help is called as soon as the child is born. Until then nature is allowed to take its course, but as soon as the child is expelled, an old woman, who makes this a specialty, is called to deliver the afterbirth, which she does by pressing and working the abdomen constantly until the placenta and the clots are removed. This person has nothing whatsoever to do with the delivery of the child. The same position is occupied by the women of the Skokomish agency, and here, also, the very best practice is followed, the placenta being allowed to come away without any manual interference except expression over the region of the womb and a slight traction on the cord.

The Brulé Sioux and Warm Spring Indians retain the standing posture, in which the child is delivered; the midwife, standing behind the patient, aids the naturally rapid expulsion of the placenta by pressure on the fundus with her hands, varied by a kind of churning manipulation.

Intra-Abdominal Pressure.—The use of the diaphragm as a powerful aid to all efforts to expel the contents of the abdominal cavity is well-known to our midwives, and we know how frequently they direct their patients either to hold their breath or to scream, as the exigencies of the case may demand; but, fortunately, they do not resort to measures quite so violent as our Spanish neighbors in Mexico, who assist the expulsion of the placenta by vomiting the unlucky patient. Some of our Indian tribes also lay stress upon the intra-abdominal pressure, and the assistance of the diaphragm and abdominal muscles, but only in case of retention or delayed expulsion, and hence we shall speak of this method farther on. The Somali of Central Africa, however, habitually give the patient warm mutton suet to drink after the expulsion of the child; this has a laxative effect, and, with the contents of the bowels, those of the uterus are expelled.

Traction on the Cord.—Traction upon the umbilical cord appears so natural, and is certainly so tempting a means of removing the placenta, that it is much esteemed by a class of meddlesome midwives which abounds in all civilized countries to the detriment of parturient women, but the untutored savage, guided in his practice by instinct and observation, is too shrewd to seek the removal of the retained placenta by such dangerous means.

Although it is customary, among some of our Indian tribes, to make a certain traction upon the cord, I am uniformly told that this is always done with extreme caution, and but very few make use of it to drag down the afterbirth—a manipulation fraught with so much danger, and unfortunately so common among more intelligent people.

The Crows and Creeks are usually delivered prone upon the stomach, and the placenta is rapidly expelled, either in the same posture or while standing; in rare cases it is delayed, and then it is allowed to remain until it decomposes, and, remarkable to say, pyemia rarely follows, probably on account of the naturally strong constitution of the race. Among them, gentle traction upon the funis is the only assistance accorded to nature, and if there be much resistance, it is at once stopped, and the placenta allowed to remain, in preference to attempting its delivery by stronger traction.

The Rus, Gros-Ventres, and Mandans are confined in a kneeling posture, in which the placenta also is expelled, but if it does not come away rapidly, with some little rubbing of the belly with the hands greased with turtle fat, the accoucheur pulls gently and steadily on the cord, evidently relying somewhat upon this traction for the removal of the placenta.

The worst practice is that of the Cheyennes and Arrapahoes, who retain the dorsal decubitus in which the child is expelled, but never wait for the expulsion of the placenta by the proper contraction of the womb, removing it at once by traction upon the cord, which will often break under the rough usage to which it is subjected, and the unfortunate woman will then often suffer from severe hemorrhage, due to the retention of the placenta, as no effort is made to remove the organ after the rupture of the cord. Massage-is resorted to, when the placenta does not readily respond to traction, and the accoucheur has judgment enough not to pull too hard. The Chippewas drag down the placenta by the cord, if it is not readily expelled with the assistance of external manipulation.

Delivery of the placenta with the patient in a different position from the one occupied during the expulsion of the child.

A change of position is not infrequently made immediately after the birth of the child, with a view to hastening the expulsion of the after-birth. As this period of labor is a short one, an uncomfortable position, if otherwise advantageous, may be readily assumed; and, moreover, the muscular effort, which the patient involuntarily undergoes in making this change, will assist the contraction of the womb. The change most frequently made is to a standing posture. Thus the squaws of the Cattaranguts rise to their feet from the kneeling posture, which they occupied during the birth of the child, with the idea of facilitating the expulsion of the afterbirth. If this does not take place within a short time, the attendant makes traction on the cord, at the same time making downward pressure over the abdomen, while the parturient maintains the standing posture.

Dr. D. D. Taylor, surgeon U. S. Army, in detailing the labor of a Sioux squaw whom he delivered, seated cross-legged on the floor, says: " The moment I cut the cord she jumped to her feet, and, standing erect, seized the squaw-belt, a leather belt about four inches wide, which she buckled over her hips and abdomen, drawing it as tightly as her strength would permit. During this time the hemorrhage was very abundant; within a minute, however, the placenta dropped on the floor, the bleeding ceased, the womb becoming firmly contracted, and she sat down on a stool looking as if nothing unusual had happened. The belt was removed the next morning, and she remained up and went about the house as usual. I saw no other attempt at expression used but the application of the belt, and this, I believe, is universal among the Sioux for the purpose of expelling the placenta and preventing subsequent hemorrhage." The Crows and Creeks, as I have already mentioned, who are often delivered prone upon the face, chest, and abdomen, rise up as soon as the child is expelled, and rest upon a stick of some sort, with the feet spread wide apart. This is to allow the blood to 'flow very freely, and, as they think, the placenta to be more readily and easily delivered.

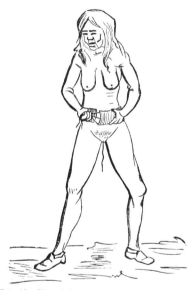

FIG. 44.—Use of the squaw-belt, Sioux Indians.

In the Unitah Valley agency, the parturient drinks freely of hot water, both during the second and third stages of labor, arises to her feet as soon as the child is expelled in the usual obstetric position, kneeling, places a folded cloth to her abdomen, and, leaning forward over a stout stick, rests her body upon it, thus exerting considerable pressure over the hypogastric region—a method well calculated to favor the expulsion of the placenta, which is thus delivered without any further assistance. Upon the Sandwich Islands they change the posture of the mother to the semi-erect from the sitting, in order to effect the speedy removal of the afterbirth, which they regard as very desirable and necessary. The patient assumes a semi-erect posture, more properly squatting, with the pelvis thrown backward and the knees partly flexed, the midwife at the same time supporting the child, as the cord is not cut until after the delivery of the placenta. At this juncture the patient thrusts her finger in the fauces to produce nausea or vomiting, which causes a spasmodic expulsive action of the uterus, resulting, not infrequently, in the immediate birth of the placenta and its membranes. If such is not the result, there is

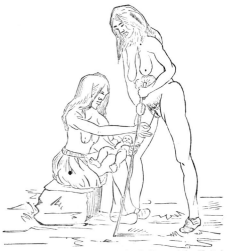

Fig. 45.—Placental expression as practised by the Indians of the Unitah Valley Agency.

more or less excitement; the woman retains her erect position, is "loomied" over the womb and abdomen, a sort of kneading, squeezing operation, generally performed with the hands by the attendant, until the flooding has moderated or almost ceased, when she is conducted to a stream or large containment of water, where she is washed, secundem artem, re-dressed, and returned to the house and its promiscuous inhabitants; children and all being allowed to witness the performance.

In Syria, some twenty or thirty minutes' time is given for the expulsion of the placenta, in the usual obstetric posture, in the chair; but if this does not take place, the cord is cut, and the patient put to bed for further manipulation. The Pawnees change the position of the patient in various ways, from the squatting posture, and pull upon the cord, evidently seeking to obtain expulsion simply by the muscular contrac-tion resulting from the motion of the patient.

MANAGEMENT OF THE PLACENTA IN CASE OF RETARDED EXPULSION.

We have already seen that, as a rule, the delivery of the placenta speedily follows the expulsion of the child, nature being merely assisted by the continuance of the external pres-sure, which serves to assist and facilitate the contraction of the uterine globe. If the placenta does not readily come, they are at a loss what to do, and the patient is often left to herself. Dr. C. M. Harrison writes from the Mexican frontier that the Indians, and lower order of Mexicans, seem to have no other method of extracting the placenta than by traction on the cord, and that he has seen women dead and dying merely from the want of having the placenta extracted. The Dakotas use most violent means, and if the delivery of the placenta is at all retarded, it is forcibly extracted, and often with fatal consequences. Other of the Indian tribes have more reason-able ways, and it is these which we will now consider. The description given me of the attempts at delivery of a retained placenta by a Mexican midwife, by Surgeon H. R. Tilton, U. S. Army, embodies many of the more violent methods resorted to. When called to the patient, he found that she had been given a quantity of raw beans, between a pint and a quart, as one remedy ; these were probably intended to swell, and thus drive out the placenta. This failing, she had been vigorously choked, as another means of expelling the after-birth. Finally, she was placed in the lap of her husband, in the obstetric position of that country, whilst he squeezed the abdomen powerfully with his encircling arms. This last ex-pedient, by the way, is a favorite method among the Mexicans for facilitating labor, the contracting uterus being steadily fol-lowed down by the arms of the husband. After all these means had failed, the after-birth was readily removed by the surgeon, upon the introduction of the hand, but the recovery of the woman remained doubtful, after the violence to which she had been subjected.

In the Laguna Pueblo, a tea made of the corn blossoms, or

the tops of the corn, is given the patient in case the delivery
of the placenta is retarded; hot cloths and hot stones are applied, and the uterus is manipulated externally with a twisting
motion, which seems, indeed, a reasonable treatment.   So
also among the Cheyennes massage is resorted to in protracted
cases, where the placenta is not readily removed by traction
upon the cord; and among the Sandwich Islanders the womb
is "loomied" over, whilst the patient retains an erect position,

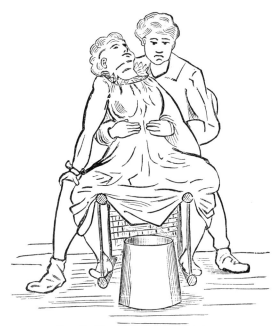

Fig. 46 —Placental expression, Mexico.

the abdomen being subjected to a sort of kneading, squeezing
operation, by the hands of the attendants, until the unwilling
placenta is expelled.   The same thing precisely is done by the
Indians of the Pacific coast, who are usually confined in a
semi-recumbent position, but in a retarded third stage of labor
assume an erect posture, and whilst the attendants are firmly
pressing the uterine globe, the accoucheur makes a certain
traction upon the cord.

A rather violent and disagreeable method of dealing with
the retained placenta is that of the lower order of Spanish

women of Mexico, who retain the kneeling position, in which the child was delivered, and drink a cupful of soapsuds, which soon produces vomiting and the immediate expulsion of the afterbirth. The Gros-Ventre Indians rely upon the same plan, but approach it a little more gradually; they give an irritant powder (what it is, Dr. C. B. Greenleaf, surgeon U. S. Army, who kindly gave me the information, could not tell), first as a snuff to excite sneezing, and thus expel the placenta, and if this fails, it is administered by the mouth to produce vomiting, and these more forcible muscular contractions seldom fail to answer the purpose. The Rus and Mandans pull gently upon the cord, and rub the abdomen, giving, in addition, some remedies which they also use when the expulsion of the child is delayed. They have most faith in the berry of the ground cedar, castorium, or a button of the rattlesnake's tail, giving castorium in doses large enough to produce vomiting.

The method of the Comanches is to grasp the womb, knead and compress it, make slight traction upon the cord, and efforts to reach the placenta with the hand, in which the patient as well as the assistant takes part. The Papagos pursue a course which is certainly peculiar to them, of producing a more steady and, perhaps, not too violent traction upon the cord, by so attaching it that the amount of force to be used is left to the judgment and the sensations of the patient; it seems as if her sense of pain were to serve as a safety valve for the amount of force to be expended, and thus the proper limit determined and dangerous consequences avoided. In the interesting description given me by Surgeon Charles Smart, U. S. Army, who was called in a case in which the placenta had been retained for three or four days, he found the attendants in great alarm 'for the safety of the mother. The patient lay on her side, with her knees drawn up, and every now and again, while he was learning the particulars of the case, she was directed to stretch herself out. The reason of this he found by introducing his hand for the purpose of making an examination; a buckskin thong, about the size of a whipcord, was made fast to the cut end of the funis, whilst the other extremity was discovered hitched around the great toe, and when she stretched the limb in bed traction was made on the placenta. The doctor found no adhesions and readily removed the afterbirth upon the introduction of the hand into the womb.

Since writing the above I learn that the Japanese, also, either carefully hold the projecting end of the cord or tie it to the patient's leg, in case the placenta should resist the simpler efforts directed toward its expulsion.

Among the Flat-heads, Pend-oreilles, and Kootewais, in case the usually speedy and natural expulsion of the placenta does not take place, the patient leaves the obstetric position, upon a low stool, and is made to stand and walk about, a proceeding which, though probably injurious to the delicate women of our civilization, is harmless and almost always successful among these Indians.

The Indians of the Misqually agency commonly use a steam bath in the very rare cases of retention. A hole is made in the ground and filled with hot rocks which are covered with leaves of the fir-tree; water is then poured upon them, and the woman made to sit over this vapor bath for a few minutes. This simple means seldom fails, and if it should, other help is called —maybe a woman, maybe a physician, if one is convenient.

MANAGEMENT OF THE UMBILICAL CORD.

The Indian midwives, as well as learned obstetricians, differ in their views with regard to the proper time for cutting the funis, but, as a rule, we find that the cord is not severed until labor is completed and the secundines are expelled; this practice we find among the Sandwich Islanders and among most of our Indians; the child remaining on the ground in front of the mother until the placenta is delivered; among the Kiowas, Comanches, and Wichitas, it is customary, after the placenta is delivered, that the assistant should take the cord between her fingers and squeeze such blood as may remain in it back toward the placenta, and not until then the cord is cut and tied. So also the Blackfeet, Uncpapas, Lower and Upper Yankton-ans of the Sioux nation do not sever the funis until the placenta has been expelled, while the Flatheads and Kootewais, Crows and Creeks, cut the cord at once, and I may here add that, as soon as the cord is tied and cut and the child is removed, the parturient cautiously takes hold of the placental end of the funis, believing that, if she should let it go, it would return into the uterus. The natives of Syria wait from twenty to thirty minutes before cutting the cord, but if the afterbirth is not expelled by that time, it is severed and the patient put to bed.

Some difference also seems to exist, and probably with reason, for the methods of each, as to the distance from the child at which the funis should be tied. The Wakamba, in Africa, use threads of the bast of the adansonia or monkey-bread tree, and tie the funis tightly two or three inches from the navel, the Mexicans some three inches. The Japanese tie the funis in two places, about one inch apart, close to the child's body; the Comanches, on the contrary, using only one liga-ture, tie the cord about a foot from the body of the child, and in Africa we find one of the tribes, the Waswahili, where the cord is also left very long and slowly dries; the navel in later years being often found the size of a fist. The Loango, of Middle Africa, on the contrary cut the cord short and dry it rapidly ; it is severed at double the length of the first joint of the thumb, or is measured off to the knee, then the child is taken to the fire and the remnant of the funis is steadily pressed by the warmed fingers of the numerous attendants so as to hasten its drying, which is completed in twenty-four hours; then the withered mass is forced off with the thumb nail and burnt (Indiscretes aus Loango ; Dr. Peschuel-Loesche, *Ztschrft. f. Ethnolog.*, 1878, X., p. 29).

The Syrians tie both sides; the Catarangut Indians ligate only one end, the child's end ; so also the Blackfeet, who, however, take the precaution to pinch the protruding placental end of the funis with the fingers, so as to prevent oozing.

Certain superstitions also exist in regard to the method of cutting the funis, a dull instrument being frequently used, prob-ably on the principle of the modern saw-knife, as bruising and crushing rather than cutting, and thus preventing hemorrhage. Some of the African tribes, the Wakambi for instance, make use of their ordinary knives ; the Loango, however, would deem it a misfortune to the new-born babe to use anything but the edge of the stem of a palm leaf ; the Papagos of Brazil cut the cord with a sharp fragment of a vessel or a shell. The

Hoopas, Klamaths, and other of the Indian tribes chew off the cord. The Klatsops, as we have seen, pinch one end with their fingers. These various procedures, now traditional superstitions, have, probably, originated in some thinking mind and good reasons have existed for their use.

PECULIAR SUPERSTITIONS AND CUSTOMS.

The Sandwich Islanders, like many of our Indians, accustomed to the speedy expulsion of the afterbirth, are in great alarm if this does not occur, and think that a rapid delivery is all important; in case their simple means do not succeed, they do not seem to worry much about the patient; the Menominees and others leaving her often in the same position for days, whilst the Crows and Creeks and allied tribes, and the Mexicans also, cease to bother about her, leaving the placenta until it sloughs away, or the patient succumbs to the consequent pyemia. The African negroes, either on account of ignorance or superstition, rarely make any attempt at artificial removal of the retained afterbirth. Among all these savage people, a certain belief seems to exist that, if nature, aided by their simple and rational means of external expression, does not speedily expel the placenta, it must not be interfered with and they turn away from the unfortunate sufferer; should the cord tear in their efforts at traction, which fortunately are, as a rule, gentle, they give up the patient; hence we see with what care the Kootewai squaw seizes the placental end of the cord as soon as it is cut in order that it may not escape back into the womb; it is possible that some such superstition, rather than obstetric knowledge, should cause the Indian midwife to make but gentle traction on the cord, and induce her to rely mainly upon external pressure, either by belt or hand, or even such as may be caused by the efforts at vomiting; possibly it may have been the teaching of some shrewd law-giver, but there is certainly some fear which prevents the women of savage tribes from making that dangerous traction upon the navel string which is so common among their white sisters; it is truly unfortunate that no such superstitious fear governs the civilized midwife.

A peculiar trait is also developed among many of these people which we are familiar with in the superstitions of some of our typical old women, who are often grieved that they are not permitted to follow their inclinations and do as their feelings and their belief dictate. The Comanches and other nations have a way of secretly and mysteriously disposing of the after-birth, so also the Loango and many of their African sisters; it is usually buried, as is customary among the Japanese; but I hardly believe it is quite as effective as that of some of the natives of Brazil, who, if it can be done secretly, eat the organ which has been recently expelled in a solitary labor. If observed, they burn or bury it.

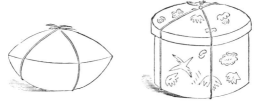

Fig. 47 —Vessels in which the placenta is buried, Japan.

A peculiar superstition is that of the Loango, who hasten the drying of the navel, force it off within twenty-four hours, and burn it, believing that the child would fall into evil ways if the remnant of the funis should become food for the rats, and as long as the navel is still on the child, no male being, not even the father, is admitted to the presence of the new-born.

CONCLUSIONS.

The same doubts as to the proper management of the third stage of labor which have annoyed our obstetricians seem to have arisen in the savage mind. We find various customs existing among the different tribes and people, and, right or wrong, they cling to them with the pertinacity of the modern writer, well satisfied with the correctness of his own view. We find the same methods and the same errors, an occasional yielding to the same temptations which beset the midwife of our advanced civilization, but in the main a correct practice predominates, and the untutored savage, guided by instinct and observation, pursues the very course which is now considered the most advantageous and scientific among our leading obstetricians.

I cannot refrain from quoting some points from the excellent remarks of Playfair upon the management of the third stage of labor in order to show how well his teachings are borne out by the instinctive practice of the savage. He says: "There is unquestionably no period of labor where skilled management is more important, and none in which mistakes are more frequently made. . . . The general practice as to the management of this stage is opposed to the natural mechanism of placental expulsion, and is far from being well adapted to secure the important advantages which we ought to have in view." The objections he makes to the ordinary practice are: "That it inculcates the common error of relying on the binder as a means of promoting uterine contraction, advising its application before the expulsion of the placenta; that it teaches that traction on the cord should be used as a means of withdrawing the placenta, whereas the uterus itself should be made to expel the afterbirth. This may seem an exaggerated statement to those who have accustomed themselves to resort to the method of pulling on the placenta, but I feel confident that all who have learned the method of expression of the placenta would certify to its accuracy. The cardinal point to bear in mind is that the placenta should be expelled from the uterus by a *vis a tergo*, not drawn out by a *vis a fronte*. . . . The distinct enunciation of the doctrine that the placenta should be pressed and not drawn out of the uterus we owe to Credé and other German writers, but it is only of late years that this practice has become at all common. Those who have not seen placental expression produced, find it difficult to understand that, in the great majority of cases, the uterus may be made to expel the placenta out of the vagina, but such is unquestionably the fact." Is this not the practice most commonly followed among our Indian tribes? And is not, in consequence of this method of treatment, the placenta, as a rule, rapidly expelled, and its retention a matter of very rare occurrence?

As a rule the patient retains the position in which the child is expelled, usually one most favorable for the use of the abdominal muscles, kneeling or squatting. Steady pressure is kept up upon the contracting uterine globe, and if its contractions cease, they are stimulated by massage, by a kneading, churning of the tumor, and aided by slight traction on the cord, the placenta is expelled. Moreover, we have seen that the Makah Indians, of the Neah Bay agency, are the only people who make a specialty of the third stage of labor; they require no assistance in the delivery of the child, but after it has been expelled an experienced woman comes to assist in the delivery of the placenta by expert manipulations of the abdomen with her hands. The North American Indians and the African negroes, undoubtedly other tribes also, have for ages followed a practice so perfect that only within the last few years the most alert of our obstetricians are in a position to compare with them; within the last decade, of this advanced age, constant scientific research has finally placed us upon a level with our less favored brethren.

PREGNANCY, PARTURITION, AND CHILDBED.

As I have already called the attention of the profession to some of the peculiar features in the obstetric practice of savage races, I will now, for the better understanding of these details, completely describe that most interesting period in the life of woman, so important, socially as well as professionally, —the time of pregnancy, labor and childbed.

We will find among the natural habits of primitive people many points of resemblance to the customs of our more advanced civilization. In their views, in their methods of treatment of the parturient, we see rudely depicted the lying-in chamber of to-day ; indeed, many a labor in the cellar or the attic of a crowded city, or in the log cabin of a secluded country district, differs but little from that which we will find in the *tepee* of the Indian or the hut of the Negro ; in fact, it is here that we often see customs which are rudely indicative of some of the very best of our modern improvements upon which obstetricians greatly pride themselves ; observation has taught these children of nature many a lesson of which, in their natural shrewdness, they have profited.

PREGNANCY.

We can trace a certain resemblance throughout ; thus a great deal of interest, and I may say of importance, attaches among many tribes to the pregnant state, be it in the jungles of India, in the wilds of Africa, or upon our own prairies. It is to the woman an eventful period of her life, and is appreciated as such by her tribe as important, not only for herself but for all her people. The Andamanese, for instance, are extremely proud of their condition, which in their native state is of course very evident to any beholder, and if a stranger shows himself in their villages, they point with a grunt of satisfaction to the distended abdomen. Among the Hebrews and other people of ancient times, sterility was a disgrace (Gen. xi. 30; Exod. xxiii. 26; Kotelman), and the mother of many children was a greatly envied woman. Conception was favored, although no laws existed upon the subject, by coitus soon after the cessation of the menses, the act being forbidden only during religious service and upon the days of the high feasts.

Abortions as a rule are not numerous; the African tribes in the main are fond of children, and hence rarely destroy them. Among some of our Indians, especially those in closer contact with civilization, laxer morals prevail, and we find abortion quite frequent; some tribes have a reason for it, on account of the difficult labor which endangers the life of the woman bearing a half-breed child, which is usually so large as to make its passage through the pelvis of the Indian mother almost an impossibility.

In old Calabar, medicines are regularly given at the third month to prove the value of the conception. Three kinds of conception are deemed disastrous: first, if resulting in twins; second, in an embryo which dies *in utero;* third, in a child which dies soon after birth; and it is to avoid the further development of such products that the medicines are given; the idea being that, if the pregnancy stands the test of these medicines, it is strong and healthy. In case the ovum is expelled, it must have been one of these undesirable cases of which no good could have come. The medicines are first given by the mouth and the rectum, then *per vaginam,* and applied directly to the *os uteri,* provided that a bloody discharge follows the first doses. For this purpose they use one of three herbs: a Leguminose, an Euphorbia, or an Amomum. The stalk of the Euphorbia with its exuding juice is pushed up into the vagina; on the same part of the leguminous plant is placed some Guinea pepper, chewed into a mass with saliva: in a few days the abortion takes place. The measures employed are frequently too severe, as constitutional disturbance, and sometimes death follows. Among Indians and Negroes abortion is now and then practised if a suckling mother conceives, as they reason that the living child is the more important and would be harmed by the drain which the new pregnancy necessarily exerts on the strength of the mother.

The seventh month is not unfrequently regarded as dangerous, as many abortions then occur. For this reason, in Old Calabar, the patient is generally sent away, as pregnancy advances, to a country place where she can live quietly and free from the excitement and bustle of the town ; and above all where she can be out of the way of witch-craft. A great many superstitions exist among all peoples in reference to this important epoch, more especially among some tribes of the Finns, for instance the Esthonians ; one of the most amusing of these ideas is the weekly changing of shoes customary among pregnant women, which is done in order to lead the devil off the track, who is supposed to follow them constantly that he may pounce upon the new-born at the earliest moment.

The same great wish prevails for a boy among savage races as among our own people, even to a much greater extent, and naturally so, as in the male child the warrior of the future is looked for ; our own Indians, as well as the Negroes of Africa, have numerous ceremonies by the faithful observance of which they hope to produce the desired sex ; but, however interesting they may be, we cannot now enter upon their further consideration.

Here and there signs of pregnancy are carefully observed : in Old Calabar, as well as in the interior of Africa, pregnancy is counted from the suspension of the menses, and the time is reckoned by lunar months ; among Sclavonians the appearance of freckles is looked upon as a safe sign of pregnancy.

The care which is taken of pregnant women depends, of course, greatly upon their surroundings and increases with the civilization of the people. We see this best illustrated among the North American Indians : very little or no distinction is made among the nomadic tribes, but as soon as we come to a more sedentary population, such as the Pueblos, or the natives of Mexico, we see that they become more considerate. No over-exercise is permitted, warm baths are frequently taken, and the abdomen is regularly kneaded in order to correct the position of the child. This is also the case in Japan, and whether the diagnosis of a malposition is made in the early stages of pregnancy or not, it is a fact that the abdomen is subjected to this treatment, and, unquestionably, in many instances, the position is thus rectified. This is done by massage and manipulation among these somewhat more advanced people, whilst the nomadic Indians of the prairie accomplish the same end by hard work and horse-back riding. The great danger in labor, and to the savage woman *the one* great danger, is a transverse position of the child. ,This they must use every means to avoid, as with them death is certain if labor is inaugurated with the child in such a position.

I have already described in full the method of rectifying malpositions as practised in Japan, in my paper on " Posture," and will only say that the process, mainly massage, is repeated every morning after the fifth month, the practitioner making the patient stand up and put her arms around his neck.´ The Andamanese and the Wakamba of Africa, many of the nomadic Indians, and undoubtedly almost all of the women of savage tribes work up to the very hour of labor. Rigby states that he finds the easiest labors, and the best results, when the women work or continue their wonted employments until labor pains are upon them; it always goes worse with those who idle beforehand, with the view of saving themselves and making labor easier. This statement we find constantly verified in our ordinary practice; we know that the working women—and we have many such—who continue their wonted employments until the very moment of delivery, have the easiest labor. It is the lady who is so conservative of her strength and anxious to do everything in her power to promote her health and the welfare of her offspring, who suffers most. At all events we shall not fear evil, and the pregnant woman will fare best in the coming labor, if she will continue as long as possible in the exercise of her usual duties, whatever they may be.

In Mexico, as the old histories tell us, the pregnant woman was forbidden to yield too freely to the desires of the husband, although coitus was indeed ordered to a certain extent, so that the offspring might not prove weakly. In Loango coitus is not forbidden. Some regulations with regard to the act exist among other tribes, and the too free exercise of matrimonial rights is often cautioned against.

The well regulated government of old Mexico was careful of pregnant woman in many ways; the Burmese women wear a tight bandage about the abdomen after the seventh month of pregnancy, to prevent the ascent of the uterus, under the idea that the higher the child ascends in the abdomen the farther it will have to travel in labor when it descends, and hence the more painful the delivery will be. In Japan, the midwife is consulted at about the fifth month, and she then binds the abdomen with a cloth which is not removed until labor begins, it being kept there so that the child should not grow too large. It is the same procedure which is followed in India, although the underlying idea is different, and three times a month the abdomen is rubbed. The Nayer women bathe a great deal during pregnancy, taking good care of body and soul. In fact, the frequent bathing of pregnant women is common also to all the higher castes of India. The Nayer perform a ceremony during the first month of pregnancy, but as it so frequently happens that a woman erroneously considered herself in that condition, this ceremony for the preservation of the pregnant woman against the wiles of the devil is usually delayed until the fifth or even the seventh month; and upon the following morning she very properly drinks the juice of tamarind leaves mixed with water.

Here and there some preparation is made to ease the intensity of the coming labor pains. Upon the isle of Jap, in West Mikronesia, they begin to dilate the *os uteri* at least one month before delivery is expected; the leaves of a certain plant, tightly rolled, are inserted into the *os*, moistened by the uterine secretion they distend, and when fully dilated a thicker roll is introduced. They are to act upon the principle of laminaria or sponge tent, slowly dilating the mouth of the womb and making labor more speedy and less painful.

A very pretty idea exists among the Pahutes with regard to the coming of the child; they recognize the approaching time for the addition to their household and tribe, and seek to make preparation for the advent of the young stranger; that is to say, they endeavor to make his journey easy and expeditious with the least possible pain to the mother. Their ideas are crude and fallacious, yet to them sufficiently convincing to be universally practised. They consider the sojourn of the offspring *in utero* as a voluntary matter, and after a given length of time, say nine moons or the lapse of certain seasons of the year, the child is to be starved out of its maternal quarters as a wood-chuck or other game is to be forced out of its hiding place; hence, for weeks before the expected event a fast begins with the mother, which becomes almost absolute as the time approaches, so that by the end of the allotted period of gestation the fetus will not only be ready, but anxious to come to the world 'in order to reach the supply of milk which the mother has now in waiting for the child starved in the womb. They of course act on the presumption that the child is nourished by ingestion from the mother. But another reason or object they have in view is, that this treatment, this fasting, reduces the maternal tissue over the genital organs and thus opens a wider door for the exit of the fetus. After this preparation, when labor has actually begun, they regard its phenomena as due to voluntary efforts on the part of the child to leave its inhospitable quarters for exterior life, and everything in their rude philosophy is done to facilitate and help the little fellow along on his journey.

LABOR.

Among primitive people, still natural in their habits and living under conditions which favor the healthy development of their physical organization, labor may be characterized as short and easy, accompanied by few accidents and followed by little or no prostration; the squaw of the Modoc Indians —a tribe which has been but little affected by the advance of civilization—suffers but an hour or even less in the agony of childbirth; the Sioux, the Kootenais, and the Santees are somewhat longer in labor, not, however, over two or three hours; two hours being about the average time among the North American Indians. The period of suffering is very much the same among the natives of Africa and of Southern India, the inhabitants of the Antilles and the Caribbees, of the Andaman and the Australian islands, and other savage people.

What little fear exists as to the occurrence of this event, which is so much dreaded by many of our delicately constituted ladies, may be judged from the instances of speedy and unexpected delivery so often related by those in contact with the Indians. Dr. Faulkner, who spent some years among the Sioux tribes, tells me that he has known a squaw to go for a pack of wood in mid-winter, have a child while gone, wrap it up, place it on the wood and bring both to the lodge, miles distant, without injury. Dr. Choquette says, that two or three years ago, an Indian party of Flat Heads and Kootenais, men, women, and children, set out for a hunting trip; on a severely cold winter's day, one of the women, allowing the party to proceed, dismounted from her horse, spread an old buffalo robe upon the snow, and gave birth to a child which was immediately followed by the placenta. Having attended to everything as well as the circumstances permitted, she wrapped up the young one in a blanket, mounted her horse, and overtook the party before they had noticed her absence.

It seems to be an equally easy process among all people who live in a perfectly natural state. As civilization is approached, the time of labor is more extended. The Mexican Indians, half-civilized, require three to four hours for delivery, and the same is true for all such tribes as are in closer contact with the whites, as well as of other half-civilized people. Accidents rarely occur; thus a physician tells me that during a residence of eight years among the Canadian Indians, he knew of no accident, and heard of no death in childbed. Another professional brother, who lived four years with the Oregon Indians, was not aware of any irregularity occurring in that time, nor was he ever called upon to perform a more serious operation than the rupture of the membranes.

This may be accounted for by the active life which women lead among these people; all the work is done by them, so that the frame and the muscular system are developed, and the fetus, by constant motion, may be said to be shaken into that position in which it best adapts itself to the maternal parts, into the long diameter, and once in such a position it is held there by the firm walls of the maternal abdomen, and the birth becomes easy. Moreover, they do not marry out of their own tribe or race, and the head of the child is adapted to the pelvis of the mother through which it is to pass.

As soon as there is any deviation from these natural conditions, trouble results. Positive statements from several of the Indian tribes indisputably prove the truth of this rule; thus many of the Umpqua squaws die in childbed with half-breed children, whose large-sized heads do not permit of their exit. The Umpqua mother will be easily delivered of an offspring from an Umpqua father, but the head and body of a half-breed child is apt to be too large to pass through her pelvis. Unquestionably this is the case also among other savage tribes.

We can then readily account for the rapid and easy delivery of savage women who live in a natural state, and the rarity of accidents from these facts: First, they marry only their kind, and thus the proportions of the child are suited to the parts of the mother; secondly, their more healthy condition and vigorous frames; while, thirdly, from the active life they lead, head or breech presentations result. Should this latter fact not occur, the mother is generally doomed, or at best, the labor is extremely prolonged and fatiguing. If the child lie transversely in the pelvis, it cannot be born, and death follows.

The nearer civilization is approached, the more trying does the ordeal of childbirth become, as in the case of the Umpquas just cited. I am told that among the women of the Green Bay Indian Agency many deaths take place, and yet a physician states that he does not know of monstrosities or deformed pelves, but attributes the misfortune to malpositions; a greater number of half-breeds is to be found among them, and the resulting disparity between the child and its mother may be a cause of the trouble; again it may be the less active lives which they are supposed to lead, and the consequent cross-births. Dr. Williams has observed that the Pawnees are more exempt from accidents than the Mnemonees, and inquires whether it is on account of the squatting posture assumed by the Pawnee women in labor; I should rather ascribe it to the more active life led by the Pawnees, and the less frequent intercourse of their squaws with the whites.

We see then certain differences and an increase of the difficulties of labor as civilization is neared. How different are the conditions upon which I have laid stress as existing among savage tribes, from those which we find in our centres of luxury! People intermarry regardless of difference in race or frame of body, and the consequence is the frequent disproportion between the head of the child and the pelvis of the mother. In addition, the system suffers from the abuses of civilization, its dissipations, and the follies of fashion. On account of the idle life led, and the relaxed condition of the uterus and abdominal walls, there is a greater tendency to malpositions; additional difficulties are presented by the weakened organization, and the languid neurasthenic condition of the subjects in civilized communities. We do, however, sometimes find in our cities, more frequently in our rural districts, strong hardy women, who lead more active lives, and who pass through labor with an ease and rapidity much more like that displayed by their savage sisters.

I can hear but little of labor troubles from physicians who are in contact with our Indians, as they rarely have the opportunity of witnessing a confinement, it is only in the most desperate cases, and hardly then, that even the Agency Physician is called in, and Indians are extremely reticent upon such topics; but I should judge from the robust health and hardiness of their squaws that mishaps are few. The most serious accident which occurs is the shoulder presentation, and that must necessarily prove fatal. This rarity of accidents is most fortunate, since neither our own Indians nor other savage tribes have any means of meeting them, save incantations or the howling of the medicine men.

The Papagos and some other tribes seem to have a philosophical way of regarding accidents in labor; they think that the character of the fetus has a good deal to do in causing the obstruction, and the more severe the latter the worse the former; hence, they deem it better for mother, child, and tribe that the mother and child should perish, than that so villainous an offspring should be born and grow up to do injury to his people.

Rigidity of the perineum has been occasionally mentioned, and in a case of this kind among the Dakotas the attending squaw relieved her patient by inserting her open hands, placed palm to palm, within the vulva, and making forcible dilatation, an assistance which few other uneducated people seem to have the knowledge of rendering. No attention being paid to the perineum, rupture is probably frequent; I know this to be a fact only of the negroes of Loango, as the information gathered by travellers does not usually extend to these subjects.

The prolapse of an arm is managed, among the Nez-Percés, and undoubtedly among other tribes also, just as it is by some of our midwives, by pulling upon it, as they do upon any part which chances to present.

Prolapse of the uterus is not unusual in Mexico and quite frequent in the interior of Russia. The Sclavonians, for instance, who are not unlike some of our Indians, endeavor to shake the child out of the womb in cases of prolonged labor; the natural consequence is that both the child and placenta drop out, to be followed not unfrequently either by prolapse or inversion of the uterus. In Russia, these accidents are so common that people are always prepared to correct them; the poor sufferer is at once brought into the bath-room and stretched upon a slanting board, the feet higher than the head; then the board with the patient upon it is successively raised and lowered in order to shake the uterus back into the pelvis, precisely as one would shake a pillow into its cover.

Hemorrhage, of which I do not often hear, is treated in some instances by sousing the patient into the nearest stream, or rather more tenderly by the Santees, where the attendant gives the patient a shower-bath by filling the mouth with water and blowing it over the abdomen with as much force as possible until the flow of blood ceases.

Whatever may be their social condition, primitive people preserve a certain superstition as regards woman and the functions peculiar to her sex. In many tribes it is customary to set apart a hut or lodge to which the woman is banished during the period of the menstrual flow; so also the child-bearing woman, as a rule, seeks a quiet nook away from the camp, or if the habits of the people are more sedentary, she is confined in a separate lodge a short distance from the one occupied by the family. Sometimes a house is erected for this special purpose, common to the entire village. Again, if better situated, she may have a separate room in her own house, sacred for these occasions.

On the Sandwich Islands, on the contrary, the confinement is more public and the performance is witnessed by all who happen to be about. The same lack of privacy prevails among the Mohammedans of India, who are as careless of the privacy of their confinements as they are of their copulations.

The wilder tribes of Southern India allow female relatives and friends to crowd around the woman, as do the Aborigines of the Andaman Islands. The Pahutes, the Brulé-Sioux, and the Umpquas conduct the abor in the family lodge, and the sympathizing as well as the curious crowd around at will. A very good idea of such a scene is given me by Dr. Ed. V. Vollum, Surgeon U. S. A., who attended the wife of an Umpqua chief. He states that he found the patient lying in a lodge, rudely constructed of lumber and driftwood; the place was packed to suffocation with women and men ; the stifling odors that arose from théir sweating bodies, combined with the smoke, made it impossible for him to remain in the apartment longer than a few moments at a time. The assembly was shouting and crying in the wildest manner, and crowding about the unfortunate sufferer, whose misery was greatly augmented by the apparent kindness of her friends. Not much better were the half-civilized Mexican inhabitants of Monte Rey in early days : but even in these cases where such publicity is permitted, men are, as a rule, excluded.

Commónly labor is conducted most privately and quietly ; the Indian squaw is wont to steal off into the woods for her confinement. Alone or accompanied by a female relative or friend she leaves the village, as she feels the approach of labor, to seek some retired spot ; upon the banks of a stream is the favorite place the world over, the vicinity of water, moving water, if possible, is sought, so that the young mother can bathe herself and her child and return to the village cleansed and purified when all is over. This is true of the Sioux, the Comanches, the Tonkawas, the Nez-Percés, the Apaches, the Cheyennes, and other of our Indian tribes.

In winter, a temporary shelter is erected in the vicinity of the family lodge by those who make the solitude of the forest their lying-in chamber in milder weather.

The Chippewas, as well as the Winnebagos, also follow this custom. The natives of the Caucasus, the Dombars and other tribes of Southern India, those of Ceram, the inhabitants of Loango, of Old Calabar, and many of the African races, are delivered in this quiet way, and the women are not only kept apart from their husbands and the villagers during their confinement, but for weeks afterwards. The reason why we know so little of Indian labor is the great secrecy which they observe regarding such matters, and their extreme reluctance to speak to inquisitive whites of these subjects which are to them enshrouded in a veil of superstition and mystery.

Some of the Sioux tribes, the Blackfeet and the Uncapapas, are in the habit of arranging a separate lodge, generally a temporary one, for the occasion, as also do the Klamaths, the Utes, and others. The Comanches construct a shelter for parturient women a short distance outside of the camp and in the rear of the patient's family lodge. This is made of brush or bushes, six or seven feet high, stuck into the hard ground, the branches intertwining so as to form a circular shelter about eight feet in diameter, an entrance is provided by breaking the circle and overlapping the two unjoined ends. In

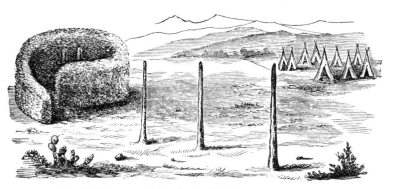

Fig. 48.—Temporary shelter for the lying-in woman, Comanches.

a line outside the entrance are placed three stakes made from the stems of small saplings with the bark left on; these are set ten paces apart and are four feet high. Inside the shelter are made two rectangular excavations in the soil, ten to eighteen inches in width, with a stake at the end of each. In one hole is placed a hot stone, in the other a little loose earth to receive any discharges from the bowels or the bladder. The ground is strewn with herbs. This is their usual mode of constructing a shelter when in camp, and at other seasons, when boughs fail them, pieces of cloth are used to cover up the gaps, or else the leafless brush is covered with skins; but on the march some natural protection is usually sought, or one is hastily extemporized out of robes with, perhaps, a lariat attached to the nearest tree for the woman to seize during the pains.

The Indians of the Uinta Valley Agency observe a similar custom. At the first indication of labor-pains, the parturient leaves the lodge occupied by her family, and a short distance from it erects for herself a small "*wick-e-up*," in which to remain during her confinement, first clearing the ground and making a slight excavation in which a fire is kindled; rocks are placed around the fire and heated, and a kettle of water is kept hot, from which copious draughts are frequently taken. The "*wick-e-up*" is made as close as possible, to prevent exposure to changes of temperature, and to promote free perspiration. Assistance is given by squaws living in the neighborhood, but no particular one is chosen, nor is any medicine-man called in to render aid. In Ceram, a temporary hut is hastily built in the woods, and in some parts of the interior of Russia a separate house is provided, as among our own Indians; such is also the custom of the Samojedn. The Gurians make use of a special room in the house; the apartment set aside for this purpose has no flooring, but the ground is plentifully strewn with hay, upon which the bed is made; above this a rope is fastened to the ceiling for the woman to grasp when in pain. The usual and favorite place of confinement for the Laps and other polar tribes is the bath-room.

As the place of confinement varies, so does the couch upon which the labor occurs. Some care is devoted to its preparation by all people, even the Susruta, that ancient system of midwifery, tells us that " the parturient should lie on her back upon a *carefully spread couch*, that a pillow should be given her, the thighs should be flexed, and that she should be delivered by four *aged and knowing midwives*, whose nails were well trimmed."

The women of ancient Greece were delivered upon stools; the large arm-chair is still at home in the East, while in Syria a *rocking* obstetrical chair is used. The Kootenais employ a box covered with buffalo robes; the Sandwich Islanders, a stone; and certain of the tribes of Finns and Mongols, as well as many of our Caucasian race, look upon the lap of the husband as the best obstetrical couch. Many of our Indians use nothing but the bare ground, others a buffalo robe or old blanket spread upon the floor of the *tepee*, or else some dried grass and weeds; in one way or other, however, they make a soft and comfortable couch upon the ground. A common method is to place a layer of earth beneath the buffalo robe upon which they are confined. Thus F. F. Gerard tells me that the Rees, the Gros-Ventres, and the Mandans, lay a large piece of skin on the ground, over which is strewn a layer of earth three to four inches deep, and upon this is spread the blanket or skin on which the parturient kneels.

The Japanese make their preparations for the coming event in the seventh month, so as to be sure of being in time. The bed which they then provide consists of a mat of straw about three feet square, on which is spread a layer of cotton or cloth. This simple arrangement upon which the patient is to be delivered is then set aside to be available at any emergency.

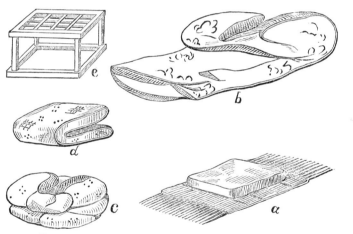

Fig. 49.—Japanese lying-in couch and supports used in childbed.

The above figure represents this mat, together with the mattress upon which it is laid, and the cushions used to support the back during the puerperal state. I need enter no further into this subject, as I have frequently referred to it, and have treated of it fully in my paper on Posture.

With regard to the *assistants* who aid the parturient woman, there is some difference in the customs of the various races. In many cases she has no help of any kind. As a rule, the assistants, if any, are females, relatives, or neighbors, and the aid they give the sufferer is about the same as that which is too commonly obtained by her more civilized sisters, the world over, often worse than none at all. Occasionally they have professional midwives, whose qualifications depend chiefly upon their age or the number of children they have borne. In case that the patient is a lady of quality, the wife perhaps of a chief, or if the labor prove a very difficult one, the prophet or medicine man is summoned. The physician is mistrusted and is only consulted in the most desperate cases ; the medicine man is aware that the forceps of his white brother are more efficacious than the rattling of the tum-tum, and, actuated by that same professional jealousy which is occasionally observed in more civilized communities, he uses his influence to malign the stranger, and glorify himself.

In Siam and in Ceram, in parts of Africa and South America, among the Indians of Canada and some of our own—the Tonkawas, the Cheyennes and allied tribes, the Arrapahoes, and the Cattaraugus, there is no class corresponding to our midwives, and the patient has no help whatsoever ; but usually relatives and friends aid each other, or there is some assistance rendered by the habitual old woman. This is true of the savage tribes of the vast Russian empire ; each village or settlement has an old crone who possesses the power of second sight, and by this gift and other similar means drives away disease; but above all haunts the lying-in room, where she causes much harm to both mother and child by her rude and ill-timed manipulations. Other tribes have their particular old women, who, for various reasons, are supposed to be specially skilled. Thus the Navajos and the Nez-Percés have their *sages femmes*, and in Mexico there are midwives who are acquainted with medicinal herbs and their properties. The Indians of the Quapaw Agency, those in some parts of Mexico, and many of the Pueblos have women who make this a specialty. So also the Klatsops, the Klamath, the Rees, the Gros-Ventres, and the Mandans.

Whenever a midwife or some other old woman assists the progress of labor, one or more younger women are always on hand to perform the actual work, whilst the midwife sits in front of her charge to receive the child. In Syria, the assistant is an old woman who learned her trade by practising with her mother who was a midwife before her; it is necessary for a woman there to practise for a long time before she thoroughly gains the confidence of the people. We find midwives also in Japan, in parts of India, where in ancient times only women assisted the parturient, whilst in ancient Egypt difficult cases were attended by surgeons specially skilled in midwifery, as it will be remembered that they had their specialists as well as we of the present day. Susruta speaks of *midwives* attending his patient, and the mention of midwives in Exodus i. 19 implies that these good women were as unskilful thirty-five centuries ago as they can still be found at the present day. From all that we have seen it appears that the *Yi* of India, the *Dye* of Syria, the herb-knowing hag of Mexico, and the midwife of the Bible are very much the same in their habits, their qualifications, and their knowledge. It is the same habitual old woman who figures in all countries and at all times, and with whose peculiar qualifications we are quite familiar. In cases where the midwife is at a loss, the aid of the medicine man is sought. The Baschkirs rely upon their "devil-seer" who discovers the presence of the evil spirit and drives him away if rewarded by the present of a sum of money or a fat sheep. Among others a priest is called who hastily mumbles a few verses of the Koran, spits into the patient's face, and leaves the rest to nature.

The *assistance* which is rendered to the parturient woman is very simple and consists entirely of external manipulations, support of the patient in whatever position she may be confined, together with compression of the abdomen for the purpose of expressing the child: in addition to this, the incantations of the medicine men as well as other means, by which they endeavor to act upon the imagination of the patient, must not be forgotten. How little actual help the lying-in woman receives, and how limited is their knowledge of correcting malposition or other of the accidents of labor, will be readily perceived if we state that but few of those primitive people, whose habits we have so far considered, ever manipulate within the vagina. I have positive statements to this effect from the Indians of the Pacific coast, the Umpquas, the Pueblos, as well as the natives of Mexico. The introduction of the hand into the vagina or into the uterus for any definite purpose is a manipulation unknown to the natives of other countries as well. At least I never see it referred to unless it be in a few instances for the purpose of distending the perineum or of removing the placenta from the vagina, which must remain if retained *in utero.* The midwife or older woman in attendance, as we have seen, usually receives the child, whilst the younger women support the patient, steadying the pelvis, resting her head and shoulders, and holding her arms and legs according to the position which she assumes. The younger women also compress the abdomen and rub the body wherever directed. The most reasonable of all their means of assisting the patient in her labor is the steady compression of the abdomen and the following down of the child in its descent. This is a feature common to the red, yellow, and black races, be it by compression of the fundus, by the encircling arms of the husband upon whose lap the patient rests; be it by the hands of one of the female assistants sometimes from behind, sometimes from the front; or by a broad cloth or binder (California Indians and the natives of Southern India) which an assistant tightens during each pain—a treatment which has not yet lost the favor of obstetricians and was once quite popular. There are some who still place a towel about the abdomen of their patients, thinking to assist the descent of the child by the pressure exercised; it serves both to correct the direction of the child's descent and to hasten its passage. In its extreme and worst feature we see this method of treatment exemplified by the. Siamese who seek to force the expulsion of the fetus in difficult cases by permitting the attendant to trample upon the abdomen of the patient who is lying prone upon her back.

All primitive people resort to expression in one way or another. The Finns, in tedious cases, compress the abdomen by a belt or binder of some kind or by holding the patient up, suspended, and shaking her as they would a pillow out of its case—a proceeding which is more efficient than mild, and serves as a last resort to the natives of Mexico as well as other far distant people. In Syria, some effort is made to support the perineum in the same manner as is usual with us. In Mexico, as I have already said, they seek to overcome the tension by the introduction of the hands, and in India the parts are carefully anointed, as it is done by some of our Western tribes. The description of an Indian labor, as given me by Dr. McCoy from his experience at the Nisqually agency, will give an excellent idea of the assistance which is tendered the Indian woman in her confinement. "The midwives, of whom there are two in attendance, call upon the Great Spirit for help in a muttering tone, and in the same tones name over the parts immediately connected with the parturient effort, and often all the joints and limbs of the body. By applying their hands to the abdominal walls they try to ascertain the position of the fetus *in utero* and usually to correct malpresentation. They use oil to anoint the parts, and just before the expulsion of the child give medicines to increase the pains."

Somewhat similar was the experience of Dr. Shortt among the natives of Southern India. He says: "When the woman is taken with labor pains, her relatives and family friends come in and crowd around the sufferer, who is directed to walk about. The midwife, an old woman of experience, rubs her with oil and bathes her back, loins, and lower extremities in warm water; if the pains are false, the woman may partake of food, but after the commencement of labor nothing is given. She is made to sit with her legs extended, one assistant supporting her back, whilst the nurse shampoos back and loins, and her friends keep up a constant noise by talking. Prior to the rupture of the membranes, the nurse places a bag filled with ashes under the perineum as a support and to prevent the clothes being stained. The pelvis and abdomen are rubbed with a limpid oil and shaken several times to promote delivery. The membranes are not ruptured; this is left to nature; when the head protrudes the nurse supports it with her hands and directs the woman to lie on her back."

Little is known to these people of the assistance given by the abdominal muscles, a help which has been recognized even in ancient times and so judiciously advocated by Susruta, who limits the efforts of the patient to the expulsive pains and advises more or less use of the abdominal muscles according to the progress made by the head of the child. The influence of the emotions is, however, thoroughly recognized, as is evident by the incantations to which the prophets of the tribe resort. In Russia, in India, and America, a sudden shock is often made use of and proves a wonderful help in hastening the expulsion of the child; it is appreciated as such by the Kalmucks who always have a number of men, with their guns in readiness, waiting near the bed of the patient; as soon as the midwife perceives the head distending the perineum she signals the men who fire simultaneously, thinking to assist nature by the sudden fright which the noise must cause. A similar practice is occasionally resorted to among the Comanches, and Dr. Forwood, who attended a Comanche squaw in a difficult labor, told me that at a former confinement of the same patient, a practical application had been made of the effect of fright. She was brought out on the plain and *Eissehaby*, a noted warrior, mounted on his fleetest steed, with all his war paint and equipments on, charged down upon her at full speed, turning aside only at the last moment when she expected to be pierced through the body and trampled under foot. This terrible ordeal is said to have been followed by the immediate expulsion of the child.

Besides the incantations which are customary as a last resort in difficult cases, there are a great many ridiculous superstitions in regard to labor, and much nonsense is practised with the view of making labor easy. Thus in the middle ages the stars were consulted. Some of the most northern of the Russian tribes think to make labor easy by obliging the parturient to give the names of such men, besides her husband, with whom she has cohabited, and he, by a messenger, informs the midwife of his own misdeeds in that direction. Should the labor prove a difficult one, notwithstanding this important proceeding, it is ascribed to a false statement on the part of husband or wife. The Finns kill a chicken and hold the animal struggling in the agony of death before the pudenda of the mother. Another custom of theirs is to ply the husband with beer, mixed with *Ledum palustre*, upon the eve of his wedding day, in order to produce deep sleep, during which the wife crawls through between the husband's legs without his noticing it. But no more of this. All of these various superstitions are equally as efficacious as the incantations of the Klamath squaw who tells the child, as she anxiously watches the progress of the labor, that a rattlesnake was coming to bite it, if it does not hurry into the world and leave its present abode.

Although most savage tribes have roots and herbs to which

they resort in various diseases, they rarely seem to make use of them during labor. We have just seen that the Indians of Washington Territory give some medicine just before the expulsion of the child, and that *Uva ursi* is used by others. The tribes of Russia use a decoction of *Artemesia vulgaris* to increase the pain; in the same way *Achillea millefolium* is used, and this latter is universally resorted to in all uterine troubles. In the government Riäsan, *Comarum palustre* is used. The Esthonians give the patient a decoction of valerian with beer. Those who have no medicines, or cannot afford them, in the interior of Russia, let the patient blow with all her force into an empty bottle, or place a vessel or pot, like a surgical cup, upon the abdomen, or they make the poor woman swallow some ashes or a few lice in place of other medicine.

We have seen that the Indians of the Uinta Valley Agency drink a good deal of hot water during labor. The Crow Indians of Montana drink tea made of various roots and leaves, the kind preferred being made from the root of a plant called *E'say*, said to resemble the tobacco plant, with a root about as large as a turnip. Small quantities of whiskey are also frequently given during labor, and so much importance is attached to this that any price will be paid for a pint or two which is frequently carried about for months before it is to be used. The Winnebagos and Chippewas give the patient, just before the delivery of the child, a drink from a root steeped in hot water which is supposed to relax the system and make delivery quick and easy. The Indians of the Skokomish agency use a tea made from the leaves of *Uva ursi* which they believe from their own experience to possess oxytocic properties. In India, it is considered very dangerous for the patient to drink water during labor. In ancient Mexico, a decoction of the root of a plant called *civapacthi*, which possessed some oxytocic properties, was given, but if the pains were too severe, a small piece of the tail of an opossum, carefully rubbed down in water, had to be taken. However ridiculous this may seem, it is not more so than a prescription given by the court physician in Siam to a lady of high rank at the time of her confinement: "Rub together shavings of sapan wood, rhinoceros blood, tiger's milk (a fresh deposit found on certain leaves in the forest), and cast-off skins of spiders." The Sandwich Isl-

anders drink freely, before confinement, from a mucilage prepared from the inner bark of the halo or hibiscus tree. Susruta advises the parturient to drink quantities of sour rice
gruel. In southern India, it is still customary to take some
food in the early stages of labor, but as soon as the pains distinctly set in, no more is permitted. Where labor is so short,
there is little opportunity to take food, hence little can be said
of the customs of primitive people during labor in this respect.

Whatever villanous decoctions the lying in woman may be
obliged to take, her labor, as we have seen, is, as a rule, an easy
one, and if we consider in connection with this the stoic character of the Indian, we will not be astonished that during the
throes of labor the mother is usually dumb and patient, and
willing that the child should inflict any pain to accomplish the
delivery. Although comparatively quiet, at the recurrence of
each pain the parturient woman will frequently utter a plaintive cry, and in this she differs somewhat from her white sister;
the latter will most frequently announce the occurrence of
pain by a sound which by the old women has been determined
"grunt," the former gives vent to a low plaintive cry, best
expressed perhaps, by the words "wail" or "whine." But
sometimes the Indian squaw gets noisy and restless in her suffering, and a description which is given of a laboring woman
in the days of the ancient Hebrews, some thirty-five centuries
ago, appears much more natural to us and is much more in
accord with the sufferings which we suppose a woman to undergo. It is said of the parturient that "she trembles and
writhes in her pain" (1 Sam. iv. 19). Her face is all aglow,
she sees and hears nothing in her anxiety, especially the
primipara cries out aloud and says, with extended hands, "Woe
unto me, for my soul succumbs to the murderers" (Gen. iii.
16). And for men there seems to be no greater threat than
"the heroes of Moab will upon that day show a bravery equal
to that of a woman in labor pains" [1] (Jer. xlviii. 41; xlix. 22).

CHILDBED.

As I have treated fully of the third stage of labor in my
last paper, I shall in no way here refer to it, but will at once
pass to the consideration of the puerperal stage, and as so

[1] Kotelman: Die Geburtshülfe bei den alten Hebräern.

little attention is paid to the treatment of the patient during that period, I shall confine myself to the *treatment immediately after delivery*, as she is then for a few moments still under the control of the midwife or attendant, and something is always done before she is permitted to go to her home or her place of retirement through the period of uncleanliness that follows.

Among the Apaches, it is deemed very essential that, as soon as the placenta is expelled, the woman should be kept on her feet, walking about for half an hour or more, so as to favor a free discharge of all retained blood and prevent its coagulation in the womb. The same custom is observed among the Dakotas, among the Flat-Heads, Pend-d'oreilles, Kootenais, and among other of the Indians of the Pacific coast, and wherever it is not especially mentioned I should suppose that the custom was at least unconsciously observed, because it is rarely the case that the Indian squaw remains abed after her confinement; she certainly moves about sufficiently to accomplish the end desired, even if it is not done with the purpose definitely in view. It will be remembered that upon the banks of a stream was the place usually sought by the laboring woman among primitive people the world over for her solitary confinement; delivered of her child she bathes in the cleansing waters—this is done by most of our Indians, by some of the natives of Africa, the inhabitants of Ceram, the still savage tribe of the Yurakere, by the natives of Bolivia, the Sandwich Islands, the Antilles, and of India. It is everywhere the same; the mother, usually with her babe in her arms, plunges into the stream to cleanse herself; or, if the labor is conducted by a midwife, she leads the patient to the water where she is washed *secundem artem*, redressed, and then allowed to return to her place of seclusion or to her home, and very frequently to work, according to the varying customs among different tribes.

Among many of the tribes of the Sclavonians, several buckets of warm water are poured over the patient's abdomen; the Klamaths steam themselves—a custom which they continue for several days after delivery. The Pahutes also continue their ablutions frequently for days after confinement, mother and father both indulging in frequent washings in imitation of some original first parents,

whom tradition informs them were very cleanly. The Siamese
cleanse themselves with still greater thoroughness, but with
fire instead of water; " with the expulsion of the child begins
a month of penance for the mother—exposure to true purga-
torial fires. It is ingrown into the native female mind in Siam
that the most direful consequences to both mother and child
will ensue, unless for thirty days after the birth of her first
child—a period diminished five days at each subsequent birth
—she exposes her naked abdomen and back to the heat of a
blazing fire, not two feet distant from her, kept up incessantly
day and night. They think the due quantity, quality, and
duration of the lochial discharge depends on their exposure to
the fire. And this is done in the following way: A fire place
is brought in or extemporized on the floor of the lying-in
chamber, by having a flat box or a simple rectangular framework of planks or trunks of banana trees, some three feet by
four, filled in with earth to the depth of six inches. On this
the fire is built with sticks of wood nearly or quite as large as
one's wrists. By the side of this oblong frame, and in contact
with it, raised to a level with the fire, a piece of board six or
seven feet in length is placed, and on this a coarse mat spread;
upon this, or on the bare plank itself the unfortunate woman
lies quite nude, save with a narrow strip of cloth about her
hips; with nothing else to secure her from a fire hot enough
to roast a duck. Then, acting as her own turnspit, she exposes
front and back to this excessive heat—an experience not to be
coveted in any land, but in that burning clime of perpetual
summer a fiery trial indeed. The husband or nurse is ever
hard by, like her evil genius, to stir up and replenish the fire
by night and by day. True, if it blazes up too fiercely for
flesh and blood to endure, there is at hand a basin containing
water and a small mop with which to sprinkle it on the flames
and keep them in check; hot water alone is allowed to quench
the patient's thirst. Those whom lack of merit causes to die
in childbirth are buried, not cremated as is the rule with
nearly all others who die in Siam. It is a custom almost universal on the entire peninsula of Indo-China and Bangkok; not
only the Siamese, but the Laos, Burmese, Malays, and others
practise it. The women of the Combodians improve upon the
experience of those of other nationalities, for they place their

couch of repose, the bench of bamboo slats on which they lie, not alongside of, but actually directly over the fire, so that the smoke and heat ascending do their full work, and they see their thirty days and nights drag slowly along, broiling on this Montezuma bed of misery. The Mohammedan Malays are as observant of this custom as are the Buddhist Siamese, so that it does not seem to be of religious origin. Sir John Bowing suggests there may be some vague idea of pacification or purification connected with it (certainly purification). There is one compensation to offset the mischievous consequences of this practice: it makes the woman of that land escape the evils that result in other countries so often from resuming household duties too soon after the birth of the child. The Siamese mother is guaranteed by this custom one month at least the fullest liberty and undisturbed rest by her own fireside." [1]

The *Binder*, which is now gradually passing away among civilized people, has its representative among some of the savage races: the squaw belt is used among most of the Sioux tribes, and is applied by them during confinement, either before the expulsion of the child or before the expulsion of the placenta, and is worn until the next day. It is a leather belt about four inches wide with three buckles. The Kiowas, Comanches and Wichitas use a broad bandage of buckskin, ornamented with beads, which they buckle tightly around the abdomen of the mother immediately after the completion of labor, and this bandage is thus worn for about a month. Some of the Sioux tribes use a broader belt, with a compress underneath, which is worn for a length of time. The Klatsops also make use of a squaw belt, retaining it as long as convenient to the wearer. Of some of our Indians, especially the Yumas, I am expressly told that they wear no bandage; and in old Calabar a handkerchief simply is tied around the abdomen and twisted so as to make it more like a cincture than a bandage; it is placed right over the hard contracting womb. In Syria the regular broad bandage is worn.

With regard to the *time of the puerperium*, or the time of rest which is given the woman in childbed, there is a greater

[1] Notes on Obstetric Practices in Siam. Samuel R. House, M.D., Archives of Medicine June, 1879.

variation among the customs of the different tribes and people than in almost any other feature of that great physiological function of woman. Some observe no period of rest, but resume their ordinary occupation as soon as they have had their plunge in the water after the birth of the child. But among many people there is a certain time of rest and isolation which is governed more particularly by their religious beliefs of their uncleanliness; and very likely some wise law-giver infused this idea into the unwritten laws of the people, with the view of necessitating a period of rest for the young mother. We find this custom as far back as we have record, and it seems that in the period of seven and of thirty days the two periods of childbed are exemplified, first that of the *lochia rubra*, and secondly that of the *lochia alba*. With regard to the first period the puerpera should be as unclean during the time of the bloody flow as she is during the menstrual flow, and this period after the birth of a male child is fixed at seven days, but after the birth of a female at two weeks.[1]

Similar beliefs existed among many ancient people: in Athens the puerpera was considered unclean, and whoever touched her was forbidden to visit an altar; even the midwife who was present at the confinement was obliged to perform a religious cleansing of her hands at the feast of the Amphidromies, when the new-born child was carried about the family altar. When the Isle of Delos was to be made a sacred island, it was forbidden that a confinement should take place within its shores.

It is evident enough why the ancient Israelites considered the puerpera unclean during the first days after childbirth, but it seems difficult to explain why this uncleanliness should have lasted seven days after the birth of a male and fourteen after that of a female child. Kotelman believes that it was because the female sex was considered the weaker, the most despised, and the one which would cause the most uncleanliness. It is remarkable that among the Greeks the same idea was prevalent.

In the second period, during the white flow, the puerpera was obliged to remain at home for thirty-three days for a boy and sixty-six days for a girl baby, but was no longer consid-

[1] Kotelman: The Ancient Hebrews.

ered unclean. We have already seen that some of our Indians seek to cleanse and purify themselves by frequent steaming, others by washing, and the Siamese by a purification of fire through a period of thirty days, which is diminished by five days for each succeeding child. According to other statements, and possibly in other parts of Siam, seven days of this fiery ordeal suffice to purify the unfortunate woman. Among the Kalmucks, a woman is regarded as unclean for three weeks after delivery, but never is she permitted to remain on her bed longer than seven days. The northern tribes of Russia, the Samojedes and others, consider the puerpera unclean for several months after confinement; her husband is very careful not to approach her, and she remains in her hut isolated, often very badly taken care of, so much so that mother and child may succumb to this neglect; only after the expiration of two months is she herself, and the tent in which the confinement took place, thoroughly smoked, and from that time on considered as clean. Ten days is the period of uncleanliness among the tribes of Alaska. In Egypt, those who are in easy circumstances remain abed for three to six days, but poor women resume their ordinary occupations, if not severe, in a day or two; in Syria, a rest of about six days in bed is permitted. In Japan, the puerpera is not placed in the usual recumbent position, but sits propped up by pillows, the mat upon which she was confined being left in place. In this upright position the woman remains for about three days, when gradually the prop behind is removed, till finally she is lying with her head on a high pillow, and at the end of three weeks she gets up and the customary congratulatory feast is given to the relations of the family. Another authority states that the patient retains the recumbent position until the twenty-first day, and then, if all has gone well, takes a bath and resumes her duties. The Yenadies of Southern India ordain a period of isolation of ten days, after which the mother returns to her household and its duties. The same is true of the Vedas, also of Southern India; the first five days after confinement are spent by the puerpera in a hut within call of the *Konan*, together with mother and sister or assistants; on the sixth day, she is moved to a shelter nearer to the *Konan*, in which she remains isolated for another five days. After the tenth day she washes with warm water and turmeric, anointing herself with oil; washing is continued for one month, when she resumes work. Dr. Shortt makes a similar report of other tribes of Southern India; he says that the woman lives in strict seclusion in a small lodge ten or twelve paces from the family home for thirty days after childbirth, frequently washing; before joining the others she has to wash all her clothes and undergo a general purification.

The Wakamba of Africa put their parturient to work four to six days after confinement. The Wazegua alone permit the woman to rest abed for fourteen days. Most of these tribes also purify by washing with hot water. The Abyssinians and the Somali use slack lime. The women of the Waswaheli sometimes insert the juice of a lemon into the vagina to hasten contraction. The Wakamba ordain a coitus about the third day, and after this the puerpera is considered clean. Among some of the African tribes the women carry an ebony staff for forty days after confinement, for the purpose of keeping off the devil.

The North American Indians seem to be less careful of their women. I am positively informed of the Sioux, the Santees, the Apaches, the Indians of the Neah-Bay Agency, as well as the natives of Ceram and of the Antilles, and the Yuricaria of Bolivia, that they practically observe no period of childbed, but go to work upon the same day or the day after that of their confinement. Other of our Indian tribes observe a certain period of rest; those of the Uinta valley take up their abode in the "*wick-e-up*" in which they are confined, and return to the lodge occupied by the family after from two to four weeks, and during this period they are considered to a certain extent unclean. The women of the Laguna Pueblo remain unwashed and in bed for four days; very early on the fifth the puerpera is washed and dressed under the superintendence of a *Sheaine* or priest, who walks out, followed by the women, to see the sun rise and to render 'thanks for her safe delivery. As she walks after the *Sheaine* she throws corn blossoms into the air and blows them around as an offering of thanks. Thirty days after the child is born, the woman is clean and her husband returns to her, but some prefer to wait thirty-six, and others forty days. A good many of these Indians, however, have abandoned the fifth-day superstition, the sun worship, and are cleaned or washed at once and get up as soon as they feel able to go about their work. The native Mexican woman remains abed three days ; on the third day she gets up and for the first time since her confinement changes her clothing. The lochial discharge is usually abundant and continues for a long time, seldom less than forty days. At any rate it is only after a period of forty days that the woman ventures to bathe herself. After that she drinks freely of a decoction of some native plant for the purpose of increasing the discharge and bringing it to a speedy close.

Very little or no attention is paid to the *food which women receive after childbirth*, yet some tribes make a reasonable change in their diet. The Kalmucks feed the puerpera mainly on broth during the first days, giving her but very little mutton, the quantity of meat being gradually increased. Among other of the Russian tribes, as I have already stated, the isolation of the patient is so complete that she is but scantily nourished and glad to get anything she can, and often, together with her offspring, suffers actual want. In Syria, mutton or chicken broth is given on the first and second days, then carminative drinks, cinnamon tea and so on, for six days, after which the quantity of food is gradually increased. In Old Calabar, the patient is allowed a pot full of chop, which her husband has prepared during the labor, to be given her, and she is expected to eat a quantity of it immediately after confinement. In southern India, the natives seem to pay greater attention to the diet of the puerperal woman than in almost any other country. Certain of the native tribes live for three days after delivery on the tender leaf bud or cabbage of a kind of date palm, *Phœnix sylvestris,* after which rice or other food, to which they are accustomed, is partaken of. The Domber give her plain rice on the first day, and on the second *chillie powder* and *curry-pillay* is mixed with the rice. Among the Kanikars the puerpera receives as a tonic for the first day a *kari* (ragout) seasoned with turmeric pepper and tamarind.

The negroes of Africa, as a rule, make very little change. The Waswaheli and Nyassa give the puerpera food highly seasoned with Cayenne pepper and other spices. The Wakamba, like the natives of the Andaman islands, make almost no change. The same I may say of our own Indians, with the exception of the Yumas, of whom I see it stated that the puerpera and the murderer are treated to the same diet; neither are allowed to eat either meat or salt for one month, for the purpose of purification. The Basuthos treat the patient cruelly in refusing her water for three days after confinement, the idea being probably the fear of too great a quantity of milk oppressing the breast. The Loango woman drinks quantities of hot water for several months in order to increase the flow of milk, and she also washes herself with a decoction of the leaves of *Ricinus communis.* With leaves of the same plant steeped in water, the genitals are rubbed and cleansed until the secretion ceases. The young mother, moreover, takes a great many baths in some secluded spot in a slight excavation made in the ground and laid out with mats, where cold and hot water is alternately poured over her and the body is kneaded, rubbed, and anointed.

Of the *medicines* used in the puerperal condition, I can only learn that in Mexico teas from native herbs are given to increase the discharge of the lochia; the same is accomplished in southern India by the use of saffron and *neem* leaves. In Syria, carminative drinks are given. In Siam, hot water has eased the thirst produced by the parching fire; whilst in Africa it is given to increase the flow of milk. Among the natives of Russia many of the stronger and more aromatic herbs are used in the various diseases, and many methods of treatment are resorted to in mammary affections, which seem to be very common in the puerperal state, as the remedies are so numerous. I will mention but one, on account of its peculiarity. In case of hardening of the breast, the patient places herself in front of the heated stove in order to warm the diseased part as thoroughly as possible. In the mean time some other person heats a woollen sock, which has been moistened with the urine of the patient, places it as hot as it can be borne upon her breast and attempts to keep the breast as well as the sock hot and moistened with urine; then some iron utensil, a knife or horse-shoe, chilled in ice, is placed upon the affected breast. The hotter and more moist the breast is, and the colder the iron, the more certainly will the cure be effected. I will not refer to any of the *ceremonies* which are here and there observed, either upon the birth of the child, especially if a male, or upon the return of the mother from her isolated state, when cleansed and purified, to her home and her family, but will simply call attention to a remarkable feature common to the natives of the coast of Borneo and to some of our Indians. For instance, among the land Dayokas of Borneo the husband is always treated badly after the birth of the child, when he is dieted on rice and salt, and for a few days forbidden to bathe or show his face out of doors; whilst among some of our Indian tribes the father, after calling his relations and friends together and having a feast of boiled dog and other Indian delicacies spread for them, goes off and *cachés* himself until the child is a week old. This practice, however, is only observed by the young men who are so ashamed of the occurrence that they go to some friend and stay until they summon sufficient courage to come back, when the wife presents the child for the first time to its father. The management of the puerperal stage by the Indians of the Pacific coast has been so well described by Dr. J. Fields, formerly of the Grand Ronde Agency, Oregon, that I will quote verbatim that part of his letter referring to this subject. He says :

" The treatment resorted to is not alike in all the tribes; some with whom I have come in contact require the woman to keep on her feet the greater part of the day, taking short walks around the camp and resting only when she becomes very weary; as a support she uses a staff, an instrument through the aid of which relief comes, as the body is frequently bent forward which brings the abdominal walls immediately over the uterus against the upper end of the stick, on which she also holds her hand, as a man walks with a cane ; for a period of three or four days the woman continues the prescribed walks, with an occasional hour in a reclining posture to rest her feet; then she is considered well. The object of this, as old women of the tribe informed me, is to facilitate the flow of the lochia ; they think that should the woman lie in bed the blood would accumulate in the abdominal cavity and she must die.

From all I can learn about the practice of the Indians here before the white men came among them, their procedure in the after-treatment was solely for the purpose of encouraging a

free flow of the lochia, and I hear of no death from hemorrhage.

Those tribes of Indians on the Pacific coast who follow a
different course of treatment, place the woman on a bed as
soon after delivery as possible, securely wrap her in a blanket
or some covering, and place her near the fire, where she is kept
in a closely wrapped condition to escape taking cold and
having fever; here she is kept for four or five days, when she
at once takes charge of the babe and resumes all the duties
that fall to the lot of an Indian woman.

During two and a half years' life among the Indians I neither
saw nor heard of a case of puerperal fever, puerperal eclampsia,
or any diseases peculiar to lying-in women. Neither did a
death in labor come under my observation; few women have
any mammary trouble, notwithstanding their being exposed to
the same cause that is a prolific source of mammary complica-
tion among white women."

Management of the Child.

The management of the new-born child is so intimately
connected with the treatment of the mother in the puerperal
state that the subject would not seem complete without a brief
consideration of the treatment of the babe. Although the
savage mother is not wanting in love for her offspring, the
treatment of the child from the very first moment is one well
suited to fit it for the hardships of its future life. Even
among those people where kindness is shown the little stranger,
where he is well cared for, and not left to starve in isolation
with the mother, as among some of the Russian tribes, he receives at once a hint of the exposure to which he may be subjected in the future. As an ancient chronicle and "Early
History of Virginia" says, in speaking of the original inhabitants of that country : "The manner in which they treat their
young children is very strange, for instead of keeping them warm
at their first entry into the world, and wrapping them up in I
don't know how many cloths, according to our fond custom,
the first thing they do is to dip the child over head and ears
in cold water, and then to bind it naked to a convenient board,
having a hole fitly placed for evacuation, but they always put
cotton wool or other soft things for the body to rest on between

the child and the board. In this posture they keep it several months, till the bones begin to harden, the joints to knit, and the limbs to grow strong. Then they loosen it from the board, and suffer it to crawl about, except when they are feeding or playing with it. While the child is thus on the board, they either lay it flat on its back, set it leaning on one end, or hang it up by a string fastened to the upper end of the board, the child and board being all the while carried about together. As our women undress their children to clean and wash their linen, so they do theirs to wash and grease them. The method the women have of carrying their children after they are suffered to crawl about is very particular. They carry them at their backs in summer, taking one leg of the child under their arm, and the counter-arm of the child in their hand over the shoulder, the other leg hangs down, and the child all the while holding fast with its other hand. But in winter they carry them in the hollow of their *match-coat* at their back, leaving nothing but the child's head out." The child is tucked away in an equally peculiar manner by some of the Polar tribes of Russia; until it begins to crawl it is placed in a fur sack, and carried by a strap about the mother's forehead. Later it is sewed up in a fur garment of one piece; for the sake of cleanliness a doorway is left in the posterior portion, which is opened from time to time as necessity demands, but the garment is not once removed or changed until outgrown by the child.

Among the Sioux, Crows, Creeks, and other of our Indians, the mother plunges into the stream with her child immediately after delivery, or, if no running water is at hand, at least dips the child in cold water as soon as it is born; salt water is used by some people who live upon the sea shore, also by the Kalmucks, who wrap the child in furs as soon as it has had a saltwater bath. A cold-water bath seems to be the customary initiation of the new-born child into the troubles of this world; it is the case among most of the Negro tribes, among the people of Bolivia, of Ceram, and of the Andaman Islands, and in some parts of India; in others, in Southern India, for instance, the child is washed in tepid water; so also in Syria, and, as a rule, by those people who are advanced in civilization.

Usually the child is bathed immediately after delivery, but

in Southern Arabia at least two hours are permitted to pass by, during which the child is wrapped in soft warm cloths, then it is washed and anointed. This is also the custom of numerous African tribes, some waiting for several hours, others performing the ceremony at once; some use fat, others, such as the Wakamba, Somal, Wanika, and other tribes use fresh butter. The Masai and the Waswaheli throw a slightly acid and astringent powder, made from the fruit of the *adansonia* tree, over the child, to facilitate cleansing, just as we use oil or fat. The Cheyennes and Arapahoes envelop the child as soon as it is born in dry horse manure, and do not wash it for several days. The Umpquas wrap it in dirty rags, and also put it away without washing. In India, in Africa, and among the American Indians, there are many tribes who bathe their children for at least one year. In Syria, in India, and in Africa, there are many who anoint the children regularly, often after every bath, and great attention is paid to the kneading and stretching of the limbs and joints, with the view of making the child straight and strong, and stimulating the healthy development of the muscles. Some strap the child or have various methods of bundling it, so as to carry it conveniently. Some, like the Chinooks, of Oregon, compress the head to shape it in a peculiar way. This method of kneading and stretching the child is well described in a paper on the inhabitants of the Andaman Islands (*Zeitschft. für Ethnologie*, 1877, p. 51). There it is usually done by the father, who warms the palm of his right hand, presses firmly upon the temples and upon the base of the nose, whilst the left hand fixes the lower jaw; then the wrists and elbows and the septum of the nose are compressed between the thumb and index finger, and so on quite a number of manipulations are performed.

It is interesting to see that the same variations exist in regard to their customs as to the *time of applying the child to the breast* which we find among civilized people. Thus among the Kanikars and several other tribes of Southern India the child is applied at once to the breast, as is done by some of our Indians. In Alaska it is customary to suckle the child as soon as it has vomited for the first time; among the Kalmucks the new-born is given a piece of raw mutton to suck, and is not permitted to take the breast for several days. Upon the Andaman Islands it is customary for any neighbor or friend who is suckling to nurse the new-born child for a day or two until its mother's milk appears. In Southern India, the child is fed on boiled honey until the third day, and not until then is the mother allowed to suckle it. In Transvaal, a soft mush is fed to the child for the first three days, and in Loango the same custom prevails, and the people seem to know the qualities of colostrum, at least they make a difference between the milk of the first days and that which afterwards serves for the nourishment of the child. The negroes of Loango hold a suckling child just as the Caucasian mother does, and it seems that the breast is only given at certain times.

As regards the period of suckling, the time seems to vary greatly, yet it is governed by about the same circumstances among all primitive people as it is among our Indians. As a rule, the child is nursed as long as the mother's milk lasts, or until another conception takes place ; at all events, the children are nursed unreasonably long. Thus the Kanikars suckle the child for three to five years ; the inhabitants of the Sierra Leone often until the child can walk ; those of Australia, from one to three years, according to circumstances ; the Alaskans, from ten to thirty months ; the Tartars and Esthonians, for a very long period, not only limited as it is among our Indians by another conception, but they suckle the child until the next confinement forces them to make room for a younger offspring. The Arabians seem to nurse for a period of perhaps two years; the Waswaheli, from one to two years; in the eastern portions of Africa, it is the custom to nurse as long as the mother's milk will last, and often during the next pregnancy. A child which is nursed during such a period is called an external twin.

For the purpose of *weaning* the child, it is customary in Southern Arabia to smear myrrh or asafetida upon the nipple. The Somal use the fresh juice of aloe leaves for the same purpose, and in Zanzibar, cayenne pepper or the gum of the aloe is applied. In case that the breasts are inflamed during the process of weaning, the natives of Southern Arabia press out the accumulated milk and cover the breasts with a poultice of soft mud or clay.

I have already remarked that sufficient or inferior *food* is frequently a source of injury to the puerperal woman when isolated during her period of uncleanliness, as it is often the cause of sickness and death of the child. This is especially the case among some of the Russian tribes. Convulsions occur frequently among the children who are partially fed with heavy bread which has been first chewed by the mother; then berries of various kinds are given the infants, not even always ripe; they are kept in a filthy condition, and take frequent colds by the use of the steam baths so common among those people. Coarse food and constitutional syphilis are the causes of early death among many of the Tartars. In Alaska, the fat of some sea animal is the first food which is given the infant. The Masai and several other tribes of Africans put a little fresh butter, which is especially prepared for this purpose, into the child's mouth after the second day. Among the Wakikuyu the child, after the tenth day, receives chewed bananas, which have been mixed with the saliva of the mother, in addition to the butter. The Wakamba give the infant, very soon after birth, a little mush, and the Somal make them take a little of the juice of the myrrh daily after the sixth month has been reached. In case of the death of the mother, the Wakikuyu and Waswaheli raise the child upon goat's milk; other tribes employ nurses, others feed the child upon mush and other food common among them. The Kossacks think wine a necessary addition to the food, even of suckling infants. In Siam, honey and rice-water is given from the first days, and the soft pulp of the banana is crammed into the little mouth. Dr. Shortt tells us that, in Southern India, the child is fed on boiled honey after the third day, when the mother is allowed to suckle it, and if the external parts are cold, five drops of the *milk hedge* (*Euphorbia Firucalli*) are given it. On the third day, it is rubbed with sweet oil, bathed in warm water, and half a pie-weight of garlic, one-quarter pie-weight of black pepper heated in a kin-weight of castor oil is given, and repeated every second day. Some give castor oil every morning for the first, once a day for the second, and every other day for the third month. From the third day the mother suckles the child; if unable to do so, it is brought up on goats', cows', or asses' milk.

The Villees, another of the tribes of Southern India (Transacts. London Ethnolog. Soc., 1865, III.), give the child for the first two or three days a preparation of black pepper, neem bark, jaggery, garlic and onions, several pots full of which are made at once and slowly dished out. In Old Calabar, the child is first rubbed over with fine sand, then with soap and water; the acid juice of an *Ammomum* is squeezed into its mouth, and a supply of tepid water follows, and for the first three days, during which it is not allowed to suck, it gets nothing but water, and later, although the mother has an abundance of milk and the child is well able to suck, a large quantity of water is given at least once a day. Every morning whilst the child is washed, water is thrown into its mouth continually for several minutes, the child gasping and struggling. This, they say, is done to distend the abdomen and make it capacious to take plenty of food, to hasten growth. If the mother is away, the child is kept quiet by filling with water, and they deem this cheap liquid very useful in this respect; although too much water is rarely taken, it may prove injurious, and possibly the enlarged spleen, which is very common among children in this country, and not among adults, may be traced to the over-dose of water.

The Kanikars begin to give rice-water the third month. The child which is nursed from three to five years, gradually, from the third month on, receives other food, but it is not until its seventh year that it eats with the rest of the family. The Vedas simply suffer the child to die if the mother's milk does not suffice, as no other woman dare nurse it, and cow's milk rarely succeeds. After the daily bath, the babe is anointed with oil and turmeric, and rubbed and kneaded in accordance with certain rules, as we have related of other tribes.

Just as adults are treated with the herbs of the country in their various diseases, so the children are made to put up with them. Teething is furthered in Russia by the use of the fresh juice of the lemon sweetened with sugar, or the gums of the child are smeared with the blood which comes from the comb of a black rooster which has been repeatedly scratched and irritated with a comb. In case of restlessness, a decoction of poppy seed is given the child after it has been carried to the ordinary roosting-place of the chickens and kept there for a while. In case of convulsions, a decoction of *Gentiana pneumonanthe* or the root of *Valeriana phec* is used. The powder of *Origanum*, starch, or lint is applied in case of soreness of the skin, and there are many other equally efficacious remedies in use, many of them most amusing and of extreme interest to the ethnologist, but beyond this of little or no value.

MASSAGE AND EXPRESSION.

AMONG the latest and most important advances in obstetric practice is the adaptation of external manipulations to midwifery: massage and compression of the uterine globe, for the purpose of exciting muscular activity and mechanically forcing out the contents of the cavity. This is of the utmost importance in checking hemorrhage from a relaxed womb, in the expression of a retarded placenta (Credé's method) or an aftercoming head, and in the rectification of malpositions (Wright's or Braxton Hicks' combined version).

Although these are recent and valued additions, so recent that they are not as yet practised by any but the more advanced obstetricians, they are the most natural, the simplest, and oldest helps in midwifery, in use among all primitive people and at all times, from the day of the ancient Hebrews and Arabs to that of the North American Indians.

Although constantly practised by primitive people for thousands of years, these methods have been recently rediscovered by learned men, clothed in scientific principle, and given to the world as new.

Before entering upon the subject proper of this paper, I will briefly outline the history of massage, which, as an alleviant of human suffering, is intimately connected with the history of medicine in its earliest days; almost equally venerable is the history of this art as applied to midwifery, and this leads directly to the subject in hand, external manipulations in the obstetric practice of primitive people. I will classify the various kinds of massage and expression and define their uses, closing with a comparison of the natural and scientific, and of the development of external manipulation in modern obstetrics.

A. HISTORY OF MASSAGE.

Of all therapeutic agents now in use, not one has been so uniformly and so consistently resorted to, and so successfully practised at all times, as massage : its history leads us back into the darkness of the most remote ages. Homer, in his Odyssey, already tells us how beautiful women rubbed and kneaded the anointed limbs of battle-worn heroes; this was to strengthen and rejuvehate the tired body, to give tone to the muscular system.

The oldest historians and physicians, poets and travellers, speak of massage and give very accurate descriptions, and modern travellers tell us of its use all over the globe ; eastern travellers especially tell us of the luxury of massage in combination with the bath after wearisome exertion or labor.

In Rome we often hear of massage. Martial so speaks of it, slaves rubbed and anointed bathers in the public baths under Nero, Domitian, and Trajan.

Thus it served to strengthen muscle and nerve, but how much more evident that it should be resorted to for the purpose of alleviating pain : we instinctively place our hands upon a spot which pains, and by pressure seek to relieve it.

In acute diseases, Hippocrates advises detersive kneading, the douche, and the anointing of the body ; those procedures which, combined, form part of the bath as prescribed for therapeutic purposes. In treating of the diseases of the joints, the brilliant Sage of Cos gives utterance to these memorable words : " the physician should be well versed in many arts, and among others, in that of massage; massage will strengthen the relaxed ligaments of a joint, and relax those which are too rigid." The father of medicine knew that by well-directed manipulations the ligaments could be strengthened, could be rendered pliable, and movement thus restored. Herodotus also gives careful directions as to this method of treating such disturbances.

In China and India, massage has been known since ancient times. The Chinese knead or rub down the entire body with their hands and exercise a gentle pressure on all the joints, together with a certain traction which is followed by a distinct noise, as is sometimes made by persons playfully distending the joints of the fingers. Masseurs wander about the streets and cry out, lauding their talents. The Chinese themselves brought this art from India; that ancient Indian work the Artharva-veda, discovered towards the end of the last century by Sir William Jones, contains a part devoted to medicine—the Ayur-veda; in this every one who looks for perfect health is advised to rise early, rinse his mouth, and then undergo a process of shampooing or massage. Upon the Pacific Islands, also, mas-sage is well known, as we learn from the writings of Cook and Captain Wallis. The practice of kneading the body with the hands was imported into Europe by the crusaders from Syria and Palestine, together with the use of the warm bath. Un-fortunately the art soon fell into the hands of quacks, but it was again brought within the sphere of medicine proper by Fabricius ab Aquapendente, the scholar of Fallopia, who util-ized it, especially for affections of the joints, such as anchylosis and others. At the same period, combined active and passive motion was advocated by Mercurialis, Paracelsus, and Prosper Alpini, who highly praises flexion and massage in his work, De Medicina Ægyptiorum, Venice, 1591, and says that in Egypt massage was so popular that no one could leave a bath without undergoing the process. The advocates of the art in the last century were Hoffman and Tissot.

During the first years of this century the translation of the book of Cong-Fou, of the Bonzae by Tao-Ssé, by the mission-aries Huc and Amiot, created a great sensation; and this seems to have formed the basis of Peter Ling's Swedish gymnastics as proven by Dally and Estradere, although not in any way mentioned by Ling himself. Still Ling and his successor Branting did much good. In the northern countries, in Russia, Prussia, in Denmark, and especially in Sweden, the Kinesi-therapie, or treatment by massage, is highly esteemed; and the names of Ling and Meding are greatly honored in connec-tion with this method. The most illustrious practitioners of the day throughout Europe are beginning to resort to it in various affections. Among them I will mention especially the names of Blache, Sée, Roger, Guersant, Gosselin, Récamier, Sarlandier, Metzger, and above all Nélaton and Trousseau, and in obstetrics, Kristeller, Credé, and Martin.

The numerous manipulations practised in massage will be best understood if divided into four classes.

First, a gentle rubbing (effleurage, friction douce). An easy gliding of the palmar aspect of the hand and fingers over the parts. The maximum of pressure hereby exercised ought never to be greater than the weight of the gliding hand.

Second, pressure (pression, friction forte, massage). A firm intermittent compression of the muscles and their coverings by the hands or fingers. The force used is measured only by the strength of the masseur.

Third, kneading (petrissage, malaxation). A methodical pressure exercised upon the muscles with the entire hand or fist in a perpendicular direction, best compared to the kneading of dough.

Fourth, functional movements (mouvements, function). Variable attitudes and motions undertaken by the patient with the assistance of the masseur upon various movable parts of the body, such as the sufferer had not been able to freely practise alone; supination and rotation, for instance.

The physiological effects are readily seen. The circulation is improved, absorption is furthered, pain is eased, the nerves are strengthened, the nervous system is especially quieted, and the physiological activity of the body increased without cost of fuel—muscular or nervous exertion—to the patient. There is a probability of a greatly stimulated idio-muscular contractility; and it seems as if massage had an effect similar to electricity upon the muscles. The contractions aroused by massage are a great factor in the process of absorption generated by it. The importance of massage in obstetric practice is at once evident. Its soothing, nerve-quieting influence allays the excitement of the patient; the muscles are stimulated to increased activity; and these abdominal manipulations will serve a most excellent purpose in uterine inertia. They are absolutely harmless, uterine activity is increased, the expression of the child hastened, and, after it is delivered, the uterine contraction furthered, and in case of atony, that is overcome and hemorrhage checked; but pressure upon the fundus, the direct *vis a tergo*, is, above all others, one of the most important factors in obstetric practice, and, by reason of its simplicity, within reach of every one. Recently rediscovered by scientific obstetricians, primitive people, thrown upon their own resources, have practised these methods at all times.

B. HISTORY OF EXTERNAL MANIPULATIONS IN OBSTETRIC PRACTICE.

It is evident, then, that external manipulations—massage and expression—should have played an important part in the history of midwifery among primitive people at all times.   First of all, it was their only help; the only way in which they could force labor was the expression of the unwilling fetus from the womb. The *vis a tergo* was their only resort; and secondly, if properly applied, the methods are unexcelled and correct, both upon mechanical and physiological principles.   I have in my former writings minutely described the obstetric practice of people, savage and civilized, in all ages, so that I need not here dwell at length upon the history of these manipulations.

There is hardly a people, ancient or modern, that do not in some way resort to massage and expression in labor, even if it be a natural and easy one.   An obstacle or irregularity of any kind they always sought to overcome by these methods.   Hippocrates, in his writings, says: " If you put a fruit-stone into a narrow-neck flask, you may find it impossible to bring it out crosswise; and even so it is with a child when it lies across the mouth of the womb."   In the case of plethoric young women, venesection was performed often without effect.   Sternutatories were given, and the nose held fast when they began to take effect.   If this did not suffice, a still rougher mode of practice was adopted: the patient was laid on her back in bed, while the shoulders and upper part of the body were bound fast, and the end of the bed next her head was then raised and allowed to fall with a jerk, which was supposed to aid in the expulsion.   Or four women seized each an arm or a leg, and thus jerked the patient up and down as she lay in bed. If a malposition existed, this same succussion was used with the feet high, so as to shake the child into the roomy portions of the womb.

In Greece, when a woman was in labor, she seated herself upon a tripod, the nurse seized her from behind around the middle of the body, and rubbed and pressed upon the abdomen with both hands.   The ancient Arabian physicians, among them Rhazes, recommend massage, firm rubbing of the abdomen in childbirth; and even now all the Arab tribes of Caucasian origin, on the banks of the Caspian Sea, have nurses to massage the abdomen and the lumbar region.   Common as the practice is in Asia, resorted to in all ages for various diseases, it was equally used in labor cases for the double purpose of increasing the force of the uterine contractions, and of causing the expulsion of the ovum by pressure.

Modern means of communication, as well as medical schools, are rapidly doing away with these primitive customs, which were frequently practised in more remote regions of our own States in the early parts of this century. Many of our older physicians tell of their early labor cases in the farmhouses of Virginia, Ohio or Georgia, where the patient was delivered upon the lap of her husband, whose encircling arms exercised a steady pressure upon the descending uterus; even now expression is occasionally practised in this way.

Among our Indians, at least such of them as are not yielding to the civilizing influence of the agency physician or the army surgeon, massage and expression are common, whether the parturient occupies the kneeling, sitting, recumbent, or semi-recumbent position; malpositions are corrected, and labor hastened by the hands of an assistant, who kneads the loins and abdomen, and exercises pressure by the palm of the hands placed upon the uterine globe. Among the natives of Mexico, of Central and South America, it is still common practice. At the time of the Incas, the exit of the child was hastened by the firm compression by an assistant's arms, which closely encircled the waist of the sufferer. Among the Calmucks, the parturient squats down upon her buttocks at the foot of her bed, and braces herself against a pole, that descends obliquely from the top of the hut, very similar to the practice now in use among the Mexicans, and the assistant clasps her in her arms, and, when labor begins, seats herself upon the ground, takes the patient upon her knees, and presses and kneads the abdomen from above downward. If the strength of the patient begins to fail, she is placed upon two boxes, and a strong man, standing behind her, compresses the abdomen with all the strength of his arms. Among the Tartars the nurses hang the woman up by the arms, and compress the abdomen with bandages; sometimes they place a heavy weight on the abdomen.

In the East Indies, they knead the back and loins—*shampoo*. In the seventeenth century, massage was · practised in

Siam in difficult labors. Hureau de Villeneuve has described this practice under the name of *Cong-fou*. He says that its object is to lessen pain, and explains it by reflex action. The manipulation consists essentially of light rubbing, touching, delicate pressure, tickling, and friction with the ends of the fingers. In this the nurse must be methodical. The manipulations must be made during the pain, and not only upon the abdomen, but also upon the perineum, the groins, the hypochondrium, and over the diaphragm. Among the Japanese, *Ambouk* is a kneading of the body, with the object of expelling the child. They also have a practice called *Seitaz* or version, in which, by external manipulation, they pretend to rectify malpresentations.

The Malays put hot bricks upon the woman's abdomen, and press upon the bricks with all their force. The Negritas clasp the trunk of a bamboo and press against it. In New Caledonia, they use violent pressure and blows of the fist in hard labor. In Senegal, some one sits upon the patient's abdomen. In Old Calabar, the woman is put in a sitting posture, and the nurse compresses the abdomen with the hands anointed with oil. Among the negroes of New Guinea, the parents or friends of the woman assist her by beating or kicking her in the stomach. In Kabylie, no manipulations seem used in ordinary labor, but, what is rare among other people, traction upon the parts already expelled is made; if, however, labor is slow, an assistant butts the patient in the abdomen. She places her head upon the pregnant womb, and clasping her hands behind the patient's back, presses first upon the back, then upon the abdomen to hasten the expulsion of the child. Some of our own Indians strap a pillow of some kind to the abdomen, and lie flat upon the ground, thus to express the fetus; others press the abdomen upon a staff firmly planted in the ground; but, as I have already stated, by far the most common methods are massage of the back, of the loins, and abdomen, to increase the uterine contraction, and the pressure upon the abdomen by the encircling arms, or by the hands laid upon the uterine globe to express the fetus.

C. THE VARIOUS KINDS OF EXTERNAL MANIPULATION—MASSAGE AND EXPRESSION—IN THE OBSTETRIC PRACTICE OF PRIMITIVE PEOPLE.

I will endeavor to classify the various forms of external manipulations in use among primitive people, taking first, as the most simple, the different forms of (I.) Expression. These are usually practised by an assistant, most frequently (1) by the arms encircling the patient's abdomen, the hands usually clasped in front over the uterine fundus, thus forming a powerful compressor.

(2.) This living compressor may be replaced by a bandage, the ends of which are in the hands of an assistant.

Another method (3) is to draw the patient's abdomen across a rope or pole, so as to force down the uterine globe. In more difficult cases (4), the patient is suspended by a rope, and the uterus stripped down by the weight of an assistant, who hangs upon the abdomen of the sufferer. And (5) an equally uncouth method of expressing the ovum is by the feet of an assistant, or sympathizing friend, who tramps upon the back or belly of the patient, or by a weight placed upon the enlarged abdomen. In some instances, the patient herself exerts the external force (6) by the tightening of a belt; (7) by leaning with the uterine fundus against a staff firmly planted in the ground; or (8) by lying flat upon the ground with a pillow under the abdomen.

II. Massage, or the shampooing of the abdomen, is a somewhat more complicated operation; in almost all cases practised by an assistant, and usually in connection with simple expression. I will merely refer to

III. The shaking out of the ovum; and

IV. Permanent pressure.

I. EXPRESSION.—Simple expression is resorted to among primitive people in almost every labor; it is the most rude and primitive form of external manipulation, and at once suggests itself as an aid to the forces of nature when assistance seems called for. It is used both in the delivery of the child and of the placenta; and the method which first suggests itself is the one most commonly resorted to.

(1.) *By the arms of an assistant encircling the patient's abdo-*

men. · That this has been so commonly resorted to at all times and by all people is evident when we remember that in so many cases the patient is delivered seated in the lap of an assistant, be it on a chair, or stone, or upon the ground. This position was common in ancient times and modern; I will again refer to the ancient Peruvian urn with the patient seated in the lap of her husband; the method is still in use upon the South American coast, in Peru, in Chili; it was common among the ancient Hebrews, in Rome, and in medieval Italy; also in Greece, ancient and modern. We find it in Africa and India; rarely among the American Indians, where the lazy male is unwilling to undertake this laborious task; here and there among the Scotch and Welsh; in various of the backwood counties of our own States; among the Sandwich Islanders; the Bedouins; and the Kalmucks of Russia.

The same method is resorted to whether the patient is delivered in a standing posture, as among some of our Sioux tribes, or among the Crows and Comanches, where the patient kneels, the assistant kneeling behind her, clasping the abdomen firmly above the uterus, and keeping up steady pressure during the entire labor. Among the Nez-Percés and Gros-Ventres, where the patient assumes the squatting posture, the encircling arms of the assistant exercise the same steady compression. Among the Kootenais (see Fig. 17, Posture), where the parturient is upon her hands and knees, the same method is in use; whilst the woman is on her knees, the face touching the ground, the hands one above the other grasping a pole planted in the ground, and the legs apart, a man straddles her across the buttocks, and with his hands clasped around her waist exercises a steady pressure on the abdomen, pulling, however, only during a pain. The way in which the pressure is exercised is, of course, much the same among different people whatever be the position assumed.

In some rare instances, in the mountainous portions of Germany, the woman is delivered suspended, in the arms of her husband, who seizes her from behind, and raises her up so that she is bent backward, her toes barely touching the ground. In this position, of course, with his hands clasped above the uterus, a steady and very powerful pressure is exercised. In other cases, as among the Brulé Sioux, and among some of the

Iroquois of Canada, the patient hangs to the neck of an assistant, who exercises pressure by forcing his abdomen against that of the patient, his arms around her waist, his hands clasped at her back. A similar method of pressure is exercised by the Japanese obstetrician in correcting malposition during the later months of pregnancy. He, however, uses his hands rather to knead the abdomen than to compress the womb, but very much in the same way as the Sioux assistant.

In the case of a patient seated in the lap of an assistant, the description I find given of a labor among the Sandwich Islanders is characteristic: It is the duty of this assistant, upon whose lap the parturient rests, to grasp the waist above the abdomen in such a way that he or she can press down upon the uterus and its contents with a considerable force, not relaxing this grasp to allow the fetus to recede. The force of the pressure is backward and downward, increased during the pains, and kept up in a moderate steady measure during the interval to prevent a loss of the advantage gained during each pain. This method is well represented by an illustration (Fig. 27, Posture), made in accordance with the characteristic description of obstetric practice in the rural districts of Ohio some twenty years ago, given me by my friend, Dr. E. B. Stevens.

This is resorted to among many of the Mexicans and half-breed Mexicans; among the Andamanese; among such of the Hindoos in India as are delivered in the lap; and among the Burmese. In case that the patient kneels in labor, which is perhaps the most common position among the Indian squaws, the assistant either kneels behind the patient, or stands astride of or between her feet, and encircles the abdomen with her arms, exercising the same constant pressure as when other positions are assumed. This custom we find prevalent among the yellow races as well as the red, in Kamtschatka and Mongolia; less common among the black, in Ethiopia, and also in New Zealand.

(2.) *A bandage passed around the body and tightened by assistants*, supplants, in some cases, the encircling arms: this is not so much the usual practice in ordinary cases, but rather a severer measure adopted in retarded labor. A description of this method is found in the *Medical Times and Gazette* for

August, 1861, describing a labor at Monterey, California: "The patient was seated in a chair, seizing with her hands a rope pendent from the ceiling. A bandage was placed about

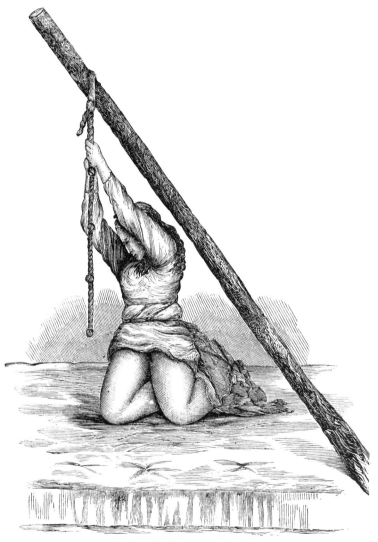

Fig. 50.—Bandage as used in Mexico.

her body, the ends of which were crossed behind, each of which was grasped by an assistant, whose duty it was to make firm traction upon the sheet, and especially to draw tightly as the abdomen diminished in size. They were particularly in-structed to make strong traction in the intervals between the pains, lest the abdomen during this time should resume the position it had before the pain came on." Similar accounts I hear from Mexico, from South America, from the north of India. The Finns, in difficult cases, when the child will not advance, force it out by tight compression of a strap placed around the abdomen; the Calmucks likewise follow this custom.

The Klatsops use a bandage only for the expression of the after-birth, and this appears to me to be a very reasonable procedure; a bandage is placed about the abdomen of the patient after the delivery of the child, thus not only aiding the expression of the placenta, but preventing the expansion of the womb; in other words, preventing post-partum hemorrhage, and furthering the necessary contractions. The Piute Indians make use of a bandage in a somewhat different way; they clasp a leather girdle around the waist above the fundus of the womb, not so tight-fitting but that it will slip up and down on the body; then, as the expulsive pains come on, three, four, or more women push the girdle down after the escaping child. They regard the descent of the child as voluntary on its part, and push the girdle down to support it in any progres it makes from time to time, that it shall not lose its foothold and slip back, and thereby lose all the distance gained by the effort for food and day-light: so as labor progresses, the child's foot-steps are followed up by this girdle, until it is finally expelled ; or, as they say, it has asserted its freedom and broken its fast.

(3.) *Drawing the abdomen across a rope or pole.* A peculiar custom, which we have not found elsewhere, exists among the Winnebagos and Chippewas. In difficult cases, more common among the more civilized Indians who have half-breed children, as is so frequently found where races mix, a cross-bar or rope stretched across the tent is always on hand, as it gives a support to the patient who kneels in labor ; but when this will not ad-vance, the woman is generally drawn over the bar, face down-ward, the upper part of the stomach resting upon the wood, and several persons, all women, supporting her arms, gently draw and push her over the bar or rope. This, I am told, is the only kind of expression employed among these tribes; an instance of this kind is related to me by Surgeon W. S. King, U. S. A., in which a patient was so drawn over a rope suspended between two trees.

(4.) *Stripping down the abdomen.* This is only resorted to in desperate cases; but, although not common, seems to be the last resort among various people. I hear of it in Siam, among the Tartars, and among the Coyotero-Apaches; and, remarkably

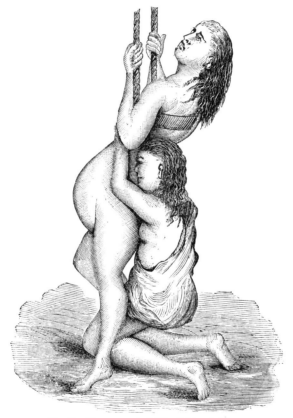

FIG. 51.—Management of difficult labor in Siam.

enough, precisely the same method is adopted in each instance (see Fig. 20, Posture). The parturient is suspended by bands beneath the arms, and one, sometimes two, of the attendants grasp the body of the patient in their arms, and strip down the womb with considerable force; a kind of "all pull together," as Dr. Reed, Surgeon U. S. A., expresses it. He says that this energetic maneuvre generally suffices, as he never heard of a case that resisted this method. That is very likely, as the fetus will find an outlet somewhere, be it *per vias naturales* or through the abdominal walls. The child must out. Other means they have none; hence, it is the best that can be done, although we should think that the mother, if not the child also, must inevitably suffer.

(5.) *Expression by means of the feet.* A very effective and not very delicate method, pursued by experts among some very primitive people, is, in difficult cases where the ordinary methods have not answered, to stand upon the abdomen of the patient, with the heels upon the thorax, the toes pressing upon the uterine fundus, and thus to express the child; or, as among the Negritas of the Philippine Islands, or the Waswaheli, among the Siamese and Burmese, an old woman, who takes the place of the midwife, places her left foot upon the patient's body, pressing upon the fundus, while she drags down the baby with the right hand. A report from Siam (Samuel R. House, M.D., *Archives of Med.*, June, 1879) states that a favorite way to expedite matters is to press with great force on the abdomen and its contents, shampooing vigorously with the thumbs and fists, and even to stand upon the poor woman's body, crowding the heels upon the front or side of the distended uterus, and without the slightest reference to or knowledge of the condition of the os uteri. In Ceram, they place the patient flat upon her stomach to force the expression of the child. The Negritas, also, are fond of placing bricks or stones, but hot, upon the abdomen of the patient to insure expression.

In some few instances, the parturient practises expression herself, either with her own hands, by the tightening of a belt, or by pressing against a fixed body. I have seen but one statement, and that is from the Indians of the Pacific slope, that the parturient uses her own hands to compress and press down the womb. How much more useful than the senseless grasping of bed-clothes or assistants by the civilized lady!

(6.) *The belt.* The belt, which is, of course, the same as the bandage, only that it can be used by the patient herself, is resorted to by some of the more primitive of Russian tribes, and by some of our own Indians, especially the Sioux, and there, more particularly, for the expression of the after-birth. The belt called the squaw belt, a broad leather strap with several buckles, is commonly used; after the delivery of the child, as the patient stands up, her legs apart, she herself draws tight the belt, and thus expresses the after-birth, which readily drops out by sheer force of gravity, assisted by this forcible *vis a tergo.*

(7.) *Pressure against the staff.* The Indians of the Uintah Valley Agency are delivered in a kneeling posture, but as soon as the child is expelled, the patient, who continues to drink freely of hot water, arises to her feet, places a folded cloth on her abdomen, and leaning forward over the stake, some three feet in length, which has served her as a support during labor, she raises her body upon it, thus exerting considerable pressure over the hypochondriac region and favoring the expulsion of the placenta; and it is thus delivered without any further assistance. This practice also exists among the Crows, Creeks, and similar tribes. The Negrita woman, who is unable to allow herself the assistance of the medicine man, presses her abdomen against a bamboo, in order in some measure to replace the expression by the hands of an assistant. The squaw of the Pacific coast, who walks about during the first day after confinement, steps about slowly with a staff, frequently bending the body forward so as to bring the abdominal walls immediately over the region of the uterus against the upper end of the staff, which is protected by the hands of the woman. Thus, the flow of the lochia is facilitated and compression of the uterus furthered.

(8.) *Lying prone upon the stomach upon a pillow.* This peculiar method, so far as I can learn, is practised only by the Creek Indians. The mother straps the pillow tightly to her chest with a belt, lies flat upon her face, and, as the labor proceeds, the strap is buckled tighter and tighter, until the expulsion is accomplished, the pressure being due, not so much to the tightening of the strap as to the pressure of the body upon the uterus, the pillow simply preventing the upward motion of the fundus. In Ceram, Loango, and other districts of Central Africa, the patient is also placed upon the stomach, if the labor does not progress, and the expulsion of the child is hastened by tramping upon the back of the sufferer, or placing heavy weights upon it.

II. Massage. Massage, by which I understand a more complicated manipulation of the abdomen—the *Shampoo* of the Indies; the *Cong-Fou* of the Chinese; the *Ambouk* of the Japanese—serves to correct the position of the child, and to

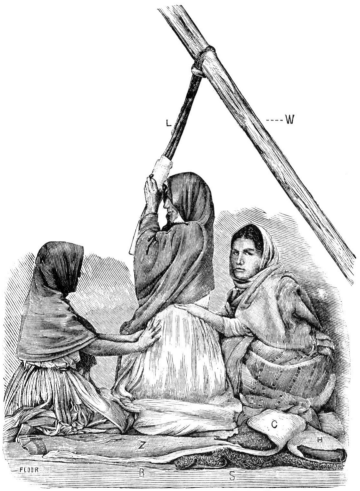

Fig. 52.—Massage and expression as practised in Mexico.

stimulate the contractility of the uterine muscles, and is used wherever external manipulations are resorted to, almost always in connection with expression. It is used to correct malposition, to produce abortion, to stimulate labor pains, but, above all, for the expression of the after-birth and the prevention of post-partum hemorrhage. These manipulations are usually practised very much in the same manner whatever position the patient assumes; and they serve the same purpose whatever the position of the patient may be—kneeling, squatting, resting in the lap of an assistant, or semi-recumbent—and they are best illustrated by Fig. 52, which is from a photograph taken for me amid great difficulties by my scientific friend, Prof. G. Barrocta, of San Luis Potosi, Mexico.

The patient kneels on the spread (B) prepared for her; this consists of a sheep-skin (S) covered with a cotton blanket (C) and a zarape (Z). Upon one end of this is put a cushion (H), upon which the patient places her head when she assumes the recumbent posture after delivery. The position of the parturient is upon her knees, supporting herself by the cord or lasso (L), which is suspended from the beam (W). Two assistants perform the customary manipulations. The *partera*, the more experienced and older of the two assistants, kneels before the sufferer; it is her business to manipulate the uterus, pressing and rubbing the fundus, at times placing one hand on the vulva, and preparing the coccyx. The younger, the *tenedora*, kneels behind the patient, pressing her knees upon her hips, and clasping the hands over her stomach, thus exercising pressure by the encircling arms, whilst the more experienced partera practises massage. (Dr. Kellog.) The tenedora assumes more active duties in difficult cases, either in retarded labor or retained placenta. She then raises the patient by her arms, shakes her as she would a sack, and lets her fall, partially catching her as she drops, with a shock and sudden compression of the abdomen whilst the parts are being kneaded. Although the methods are very much the same among all people and in all positions, slight differences are here and there observed; for instance, among the Papagos, one of the assistants places herself in a kneeling posture behind the patient, with one knee pressing upon the lumbar region, while she grasps the body of the sufferer with both hands immediately under the ribs in front. The other assistant places herself in a kneeling position in front of the patient, and with the palms of her hands rubs the abdomen thoroughly, the pressure being constantly exercised downwards from the spine of the ilium to the pubis. They appreciate the differ-

ence between primipara and multipara, and with the former
they do not resort to the same degree of pressure and friction as in the multipara, being evidently aware of the more
firm tone of the abdominal muscles, and of the longer time
needed. In Africa and in India, we find not unfrequently that
warmth and oil aid in this process, as among the Gros-Ventres, where the assistant greases her hands with turtle fat and
warms them over the hot embers, and quickly applying the
heated hands to the patient's abdomen, rubs and presses it downward and backward. These manipulations are, of course,
more readily practised with the patient in a kneeling or squatting position, and especially when seated semi-recumbent in
the lap of an assistant, whose encircling arms afford the means
of compression. But with the necessary variations, it is the
same whatever position the patient assumes. For instance,
among the Hoopa, Klamath, or Penemone Indians, the patient
lies down in a semi-recumbent position, whilst an assistant
kneels at either side, rubbing and pressing the abdomen. So,
also, among the Siamese, where the patient is on her back, a
woman takes position on either side, and they begin by forcibly pressing the abdomen backward and down for three to five
hours, and, if then they fail to expel the fetus, one tramps
upon the abdomen, and, as we have learned, if this does not
succeed, the more forcible method of suspension is resorted to.
Instead of the hands, the thumbs and fists are used by some.
For instance, as in Siam, where they shampoo the abdomen
vigorously in this method, stroking and pressing it downward
at the same time. Among some people I find no reference to
the use of massage, but have considered this more as an omis-
sion upon the part of my informants. For instance, among
the Chippewas and Blackfeet, lower and upper Yanktonais,
nothing is said of the use of massage by my correspondent.
So, also, among the Santees and Dakotas, the Cherokees, Choc-
taws, Chicasaws, Seminoles, Cheyennes, Arapahoes, Assne-
boines. It is, however, an almost universal agent, and, whether
among our own Indians, the Mexicans, or natives of South
America, the Vedas of India, the ancient Ainos, or the
modern Japanese, the inhabitants of the Caucasus, or of the
Himalayas, of the Australian Islands, or of Africa, we find that

massage is everywhere the main and almost the only reliance in labor.

III. SHAKING UP OF THE PATIENT.—Though not strictly within the sphere of this paper, I will briefly refer to some of those peculiar and barbarous methods to which these primitive people resort in their despair. We have already observed how, in Mexico, the tenedora raises the patient up and drops her, catching her with a shock so as to shake out the uterine contents, shaking out the child from the womb as she would flour out of a sack. In Southern India, they shake her several times to promote delivery, but, if this does not answer, they roll the patient upon the ground, or suspend her by her feet and shake her several times. The object of this is, evidently, after they have seen that the child cannot be expelled in the natural way, to throw the fetus out of the pelvis proper into the roomier upper portion, so that it may change its position, and come with head or breech first. We find a precisely similar custom among the Nez-Percés Indians, who take the patient, if labor is prolonged, reverse her, and whilst the head rests upon the ground, shake the body vigorously in the air; then they lead her to a stake again and see if the condition of affairs is at all improved; if not, the process is again repeated. This they do several times, and, if finally it proves of no avail, the midwife introduces her hand, and pulls at whatever she can reach. If it happens to be a foot, well and good; if it happens to be an arm, the patient will probably be so injured that death results, as my correspondent tells me he has never heard of a woman surviving the graver accidents of parturition. The Esthonians hold the patient in the air, shaking her vigorously if labor is retarded. In Syria, the patient is rolled in a blanket if she is not confined within twenty-four hours after the commencement of labor, and four male or female friends seize the corners of the blanket and roll the poor woman about in various directions, and bounce her up and down to facilitate confinement.

IV. PERMANENT PRESSURE.—Bandages of cloth or leather, ropes or belts, are occasionally resorted to, but are not found as often as in the lying-in room of civilization. They are used here and there in pregnancy, labor, and child-bed. In pregnancy, the binder is used in Japan from about the fifth month on to prevent the growth of the child, so that it may not become too'large, and delivery may be easy. In India and in Burmah, as well as among one or two of our own Indian tribes, the bandage is used, tightly worn, after the seventh month, in order that the uterus may not ascend too high, that the child may not have so far to go when it wishes to escape. In labor, the simple binder is rarely resorted to. Usually when the binder is applied, it serves as an active means of compression; but among one of the Indian tribes, as we have seen, the simple belt is used, which is pressed down so as to follow the uterus with each pain. In child-bed, or rather in the time following delivery, as the bed is but rarely resorted to, the binder plays a very insignificant part. We have seen, especially among the Sioux, the squaw belt used, but it is worn for only, perhaps, twelve hours after labor. In Mexico, a tight bandage is sometimes used, or a rope. In Old Calabar, a simple handkerchief answers the purpose. The Kiowas, Comanches, and several other Indian tribes use it; but whether travellers or other authorities who have written upon the subject neglected to mention the binder or not, I rarely hear of it.

D. THE USES OF MASSAGE AND EXPRESSION.

In speaking of the different kinds of external manipulations and the various methods of applying them, we have naturally spoken to some extent of the purposes for which they are used. But it may be well to consider these somewhat more in detail, and I will endeavor to describe the various purposes served by these external manipulations in pregnancy, labor, and in childbirth.

I. PREGNANCY.—Steady pressure, as we have seen, is used to prevent the undue growth of the ovum ; but massage properly is resorted to for the purpose (1) *of correcting malpositions.* Thus, in Japan, the medicine-man manipulates the abdomen of the patient, who clings about his neck, pressing his shoulders against her breasts, and pressing his knees between hers, so that she is firmly supported. Then he practises a lateral massage with his hands, beginning at the seventh cervical vertebra, and rubbing downward and forward, rubbing also the nates and hips with the palms of his hands, repeating the movement from sixty to seventy times every morning after the fifth month. This, I judge, is only in case of wealthy or handsome patients, or when malpositions are expected for certain superstitious reasons. By far more frequently is massage used for the purpose (2) of producing *abortion.* Among some of our own Indians, the Piutes among others, many of the natives of Australia, the inhabitants of the Sierra Leone, and of the interior of Africa, the Loango negroes, and others, produce abortion, either by firmly kneading and rubbing the abdomen with the hands, or pounding and working it with their fists. Many do it for criminal purposes, others because they dread the often fatal labor with half-breed children. This is a somewhat remarkable circumstance, but true among our own Indians upon the Pacific Coast and in the interior, in Australia, and in India, that labor following intercourse with whites is always tedious and dangerous, frequently ending in the death of both mother and child. Hence they produce abortion in preference to undergoing this ordeal. In India and in Africa, abortion is often produced when the mother is suckling one infant and finds herself pregnant with another.

II. Labor.—Massage in (1) *normal labor* is almost invariably used unless the case be a very simple and rapid one, or the poor sufferer be without friends and means. It serves the purpose of improving or correcting the position of the child, of stimulating the uterine contractions, and of directly aiding by mechanical pressure the muscular action. A slight variation, ordinary flexion and pressure upon the abdomen, regular massage, combined with expression, is used in ordinary cases.

(2.) *Malposition.*—In cases of malposition, which are only discovered by the simple fact that the child is not expelled in proper time, more violent means are resorted to, such as forcible kneading, shaking, tossing in a blanket, and tramping upon the abdomen. Thus, by violent means, there is a possibility of forcing the child into its proper axis, with breech or head in the pelvis, and this done, of forcing it out through the natural passages. These external manipulations are, as we have seen, their only resort; and as death is the consequence of an undelivered child, every means in their power must be taken to expel it; and these very forcible means must almost inevitably force a rupture somewhere. If the child is not crowded out through the natural outlet, a place of least resistance will be found elsewhere; the womb or abdominal walls must give way. The child must out or the patient must die.

(3.) *Placenta.* The placenta usually follows the child, but unless this is the case, massage and expression are invariably resorted to. Frequently the patient retains the same position which she assumed during labor, and the attendants continue the same manipulations until the after-birth is expelled. Rarely does she assume a different position, as among the Sioux, where the squaw belt is used, the parturient jumps up after the delivery of the child, draws tight her belt, and thus forces out the placenta. Then, again, others press with the abdomen against a staff fast in the ground. In short, the milder means of massage and expression are used in this stage of labor by the various people. It may be again remarked that primitive people, odd as it may seem, rarely pull upon the cord, but in most instances use the *vis a tergo*, stimulate the activity of the womb by friction of the fundus, and press out the contents. Massage, combined with expression of various kinds, never very forcible, is used in this stage of labor.

III. CHILD-BED. I have not found any reference to the use of massage after the expulsion of the placenta. Expression, of course, does not come in question; but permanent pressure, as we have already seen, is occasionally used. I will not here again refer to it, as being really foreign to our subject. In some few instances, as among certain tribes upon the Pacific coast, some pressure is at times exercised upon the abdomen during the first day after confinement, the patient walking about, occasionally stops to lean with the abdomen upon a staff, and the compression of the uterus forces out the discharge. Among some of the Indian tribes, but especially among the natives of Africa and India, the infant is thoroughly kneaded and massaged after each bath; and this very excellent procedure undoubtedly serves to strengthen the tender muscles.

E. THE DEVELOPMENT OF EXTERNAL MANIPULATION IN RECENT OBSTETRIC PRACTICE.

The use of external manipulation in child-birth is, as we have seen, a most ancient and venerable practice, forgotten by civilization for ages, and only of late years again accorded the importance which simple-minded, primitive people have always conceded to it.

Phélippeaux, in his "Etude Pratique sur les Frictions et le Massage," Paris, 1870, justly says: Within a few years, in the presence of numerous well-authenticated and, we may almost say, marvellous facts, a return has been brought about to a legitimate and long-forgotten practice. To-day the most illustrious masters look kindly upon a method of treatment as old as the world, which has now been deprived of the surrounding fables and charlatanism. The use of external manipulations in obstetric practice has rapidly advanced in importance in the course of this century. In 1812, Wigand discovered the important fact that, by the aid of external pressure, malpositions could be corrected; but his views, although addressed to the academies of Berlin and Paris, were neglected and forgotten: yet he had only stated distinctly what Hippocrates had vaguely indicated, and what Jacob Rueffius and Mercurius Scipio had urged. The Hamburg obstetrician was forgotten until 1859, when the translation of his work by Belin and Hergott appeared in Strasburg. This was taken up by Stoltz and Cazeaux. Then comes Wright, of Cincinnati, and, soon after, Braxton Hicks, to whom the credit has so long been unjustly given; and in 1853 and in 1860, Credé, who so earnestly advocated delivery by means of expression, endeavoring to imitate nature as nearly as possible by provoking uterine contractions, forcing the descent by a *vis a tergo*, the hand never touching the genitals of the patient, the entry of air, as well as traumatism, were impossible. Credé's method was already indicated by Busch in 1803. Then, in 1867, comes Kristeller, advocating uterine expression for the delivery of the child itself; and, in 1865, Martin, of Berlin, attempted to obtain the after-coming head by means of manual expression after the delivery of the body. Although Credé's method is so perfectly natural, simple in principle, and easy in application, it has yet but slowly asserted itself. Even in Germany, among his immediate surroundings, it was a long time before the method gained ground. (L'Expression Utérine, A. T. Suchard, Paris, 1872.) In 1856, von Ritgen urged that the forceps should never be used without the accompanying aid of manual expression, and Seyfert, of Prague, pointed out the merits of these methods at every possible opportunity, on account of his great aversion to all such methods of delivery which necessitated the introduction of hand or instrument into the genital tract. He sought to obtain the delivery of the uterine contents as does nature herself, by pressure from above, not by traction from below.

Massage and expression being the only resort in the hands of primitive people for the completion of difficult labor, they intuitively, by instinct and by long practice, not by scientific reasoning, of course, have brought them to a certain state of perfection, although brute force is more relied upon than dexterous manipulation. The methods are so simple, so natural, and so thoroughly in accordance with sound mechanical principles, that they have produced good results. Deprived of the brutality of physical force and aided by science, these very means which have so long and so well served the ignorant will attain a high degree of perfection, and will serve by far better the scientific obstetrician.

LITERATURE.

I have not here referred to my authorities, as I have, in my earlier papers, given due credit to the numerous professional brethren who have so kindly and so indefatigably aided me in my work. I have compiled the facts here given from the same data; *i. e.*, information gathered from individual friends, from the letters received from the Surgeons of the U. S. A., and from the Agency Physicians in response to the circular letter of inquiry, sent by Major Powell, of the Bureau of Ethnology of the Smithsonian Institution; from medical works and the reports of travellers, especially the Zeitschrift für Ethnologie, and the following books and papers, bearing more particularly upon massage. From the first three I have drawn largely; of the last three I have only seen extracts.

A. F. SUCHARD : De l'Expression Utérine Appliqué au Fœtus. Paris, 1872.

LE DR. PHÉLIPPEAUX : Etude Pratique sur les Frictions et le Massage. Paris, 1870.

DR. BELA WEISS: Die Massage, ihre Geschichte, ihre Anwendung und Wirkung. Wiener Klinik, xi. u. xii., Nov. and Dec., 1879.

DR. J. ESTRADÈRE. Paris, 1863.

SAVARY: Etude Pratique sur les Frictions et le Massage, par M. LE DR. PHÉLIPPEAUX. Paris. Delahaye, p. 116.

R. KREBEL : Volksmedizin u. Volksmittel verschiedener Völkerstämme Russlands. Leipzig et Heidelberg, 1858.

HUREAU DE VILLENEUVE : De l'Accouchement dans la race Jaune. Thèse de Paris, 1863.

MALLAT : Les Phillipines. Paris, 1826.

DR. LECLERC : Une Mission Médicale en Kabylie. Paris, 1846.

MOSENGEIL : Archiv f. klin. Chirurgie, 19, p. 551.

GERST : Ueber den therapeutischen Werth der Massage. Würzburg, 1879.

CREDÉ : Monatsschrift f. Geburtsk., vol. xvi., p. 274, 1861.

MUNDÉ, P. F.: Palpation in Obstetrics. AM. JOUR. OBSTET., October, 1879, and April, 1880

CHARACTERISTIC LABOR SCENES

AMONG THE YELLOW, BLACK, AND RED RACES.

A S I have described the posture of women and the methods of treatment habitual among various people in the different stages of labor, I will now relate individual labor scenes among Mongolians, Indians and Negroes, which may be regarded as typical, so far as that is possible. And these will, I trust, serve for the better understanding of the peculiarities in the management of childbirth as customary among these races.

MONGOLIANS.

The Japanese and the Ainos, the aborigines of Japan, as well as the Kalmucks, must serve as a type of the yellow races: the obstetric customs of the former are so well described by my friend Dr. J. C. Cutter, of Kaita Kaschi, Lappou, Japan, in his kind response to my circular letter, that I can do no better than follow him *verbatim*, after picturing the treatment of the pregnant woman as detailed to me by Dr. N. Kauda, of Tokio.

JAPANESE.

Dr. Kauda says: " During the fifth month after conception the pregnant woman first consults a midwife, who binds her abdomen with a band of cloth, one foot wide and six and one-half feet long, which is never removed until the delivery of the child, although occasionally changed. This binding of the abdomen is for the purpose of preventing the growth of the child, in order that delivery may be made easy. About three times a month the midwife comes to rub the abdomen, and in the seventh month preparations are made for the approaching labor."

In reference to the present inhabitants of Japan, Dr. Cutter says :

" With regard to the assistants who attend the parturient woman, I may state that it is very rare that a man is present during confinement; the lady (or coolie-woman) is assisted in her labor by a *samba-san*—i. e., a female in reduced circumstances. Usually this is not an educated midwife, but some elderly woman, or widow, who has been taught her duties by a former *samba-san*.

"At present there is a school at Tokio for the education of midwives ; and at all of the hospitals in the empire instruction can be secured from the medical officers of the same, by women desirous of becoming midwives. The ' Home Department Instructions,' issued in the 9th year of Meiji (1876) contains the following :

" 'ART. 2. Anyone desirous to become an obstetrician, oculist or dentist, can obtain a license after he or she has satisfactorily passed an examination in the general principles of anatomy and physiology, and in the pathology of such parts of the body as he or she has to treat.'

" Such is the regulation ; in Tokio its provisions may be insisted upon—in other parts of the empire I have doubts about its enforcement.

" The Japanese women are healthy, well formed, and well developed, as they have not been injured by the fashionable-torture apparatuses in use in Europe and America. Hence, in the majority of the cases, the *samba-san* has only to receive the child and to remove the placenta. The Japanese females all have roomy pelves, and naturally they do not look forward with dread to their confinement, having, moreover, implicit confidence in the powers of nature to do all that will be required in their case.

" When the time of confinement approaches, a thick, padded *futon* (i. e., a thin, cotton-filled mattress) is placed on the *tatamé* or straw matting. At one end a number of *futon* are rolled up and used as cushions, against which the parturient reclines, occupying the usual Japanese posture, i. e., as in the illustration. The knees are bent, the legs under the thighs, and to the outside, the toes outwards; the knees are separated during the delivery of the child. Before the patient are often placed a pile of *futon* or a chair or

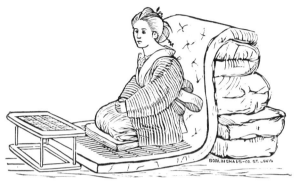

Fig. 53.

peculiar stool, against which she leans; in other cases a female friend takes the usual posture in front of her, and another behind her to support the weary body, to hold her head, and even to exert a hugging pressure about the abdomen. The *samba-san* rubs the abdomen, lightly percusses it, and even exerts pressure. Later she receives the child as it presents and holds it up while being expelled. The uterus is not followed down by abdominal pressure.

"The placenta is obtained in the same posture; in almost all cases the *samba-san* puts two loops on the cord, severs it and waits for the placenta to appear. Occasionally she uses traction and abdominal pressure. After this a thick sash, or *obé*, is wound several times about the body, and the mother then reclines upon the *futon*.

"During pregnancy, the ladies avoid unpleasant sights, sounds and conversations. They will not eat of rabbit or hare, willingly, for fear of the production of 'hare-lip:' in some provinces they will eat no flesh during this period, in others, during the last twenty-one days of the pregnancy, the woman withdraws to a separate room—a wealthy lady to a separate house. This seclusion is continued for twenty-one days after delivery; then she also has food prepared apart from that of the remainder of the household.

"Before confinement additional religious duties are not often undertaken : the patient rarely makes special visits to the temple, rarely enlarges her charitable duties. She merely takes several baths, changes all her garments, sets aside changes of under-wear, and now patiently and quietly awaits the workings of nature.

"After labor, as we should say during the period of child-bed, the Japanese mother keeps to her house twenty-one days. On the seventh day, if all is favorable, or later, on the twenty-first day after delivery, a dinner is given to all the relatives. If it is a boy, there are then great rejoicings and long-drawn out wordy congratulations; if a girl, all expressions are severely moderated.

"If a girl, on the thirty-first day, if a boy, on the fiftieth day, the mother, the child, and special female friends go to the temple. The *Bonze* recites special prayers, and gives the mother a special protecting prayer written on the temple paper, which is many times folded and then deposited in a girdle-bag.

"Some peculiar customs are observed with regard to the after-birth : the umbilical cord is severed from the pla-centa, wrapped in several thicknesses of white paper, then in a paper containing the father's and mother's names in full. Thus prepared it is laid aside with the family archives. If the child dies, it is buried with him; if he lives to adult age, he constantly carries it about with him, and at last it is buried with him.

"The placenta itself is taken from the room in an established form of earthen vessel: if it is a boy's, a stick of India ink and a writing brush are placed with it; if a girl's, nothing. In either case, the placenta is buried deep in the earth, beyond the reach of dogs."

THE KARAFUTO AINOS, OF ISCHARI VALLEY OF HOKKAIDO (YEZO).

"Among these people, the original inhabitants and rulers of Japan, the parturient is assisted by an elderly female, who has had several children but is not specially instructed for her office, nor especially selected for her intelligence. Other females, at times, come to the hut, but take no active part. If the labor is much delayed, and the woman becomes exhausted, her husband is called in to help support her; the priest is sent for, to prepare some white sticks, which are shaved down from one end to form an object not unlike a New England split wood broom, whose fibers have not been bent back to be confined by the cord; these latter are stuck into the ground about the hut, leaving the frayed edges upper-most. If an arm or a leg presents, the fetus, whole or part, is pulled away by sheer force, usually with fatal result, not only to the fetus, but to the mother. Their resorts in difficult cases are very limited, and it is not infrequent for the mother to perish from hemorrhage. The only instrument in use is a thong or cord for traction during impaction or mal-presentation.

"As the Ainos *meuoki* not only spins and weaves the tree-fibers, but aids in hunting, fishing, bearing burdens and drawing loads, she is usually of a strong, vigorous frame, and of excellent development. She possesses a roomy pelvis with well proportioned adjuncts, and rarely suffers from disease, excepting syphilis, parasites, and occasional indigestion from gluttony.

"*Position.*—The houses in which the people live are very rude; sometimes a cave in the hill-side, with a hole in the roof for smoke; more often, a rude pole structure, thatched on roof and sides with long wild grass. In the center of the one large room is an open fire; at one end of the room may be a narrow board floor; around the sides are collections of straw and old garments, upon which men, women, children and dogs sleep promiscuously. The wealthy ones have a few blankets, an occasional *futon*, and now and then a *tatamé*. The majority live in a very wretched manner.

"Scanty preparations are made for approaching labor; shortly before full time the expectant mother gathers a small amount of a peculiar fine white grass, which is carefully dried, and, on the day of the delivery, spread out on the floor or ground on one side of the fire. During the early part of the labor she attends to simple duties, or reclines at pleasure on the straw or mats. At the onset of active labor pains she approaches the fire, drops on her knees, then separates them, and rests back on her heels, while her toes are extended outwards. The midwife faces her; between them a rope with knots or cross sticks is suspended from the roof. This is seized by the parturient, who pulls lustily upon it. The midwife helps to sustain her in this position. The child is dropped on the straw between the mother's legs, and is not molested until the placenta appears. A noose is put about the cord, when the latter is cut. The midwife takes up the child, and spurts a mouthful of cold water upon its chest; if it screams lustily it is a good child, otherwise, not much is thought of it.

"*Placenta.*—The patient remains in her position, and the placenta usually appears in a short time; if not, the old woman pulls it out. From this latter procedure, hemorrhages are not infrequent. I have yet to learn that massage or pressure is used at this stage. A tree-fiber girdle is now assumed outside of the usual *kimono*, or flowing garment.

"The labor generally lasts from eight to forty-eight hours. The child is not washed, but is wrapped up in an old *momu* (a cloth made of the inner fibers of a yezo tree): it is allowed to suckle from three to five years, and even longer, and is carried about on its nurse's back under the outer garments and next to the skin.

" They have no obstetrical instruments. Abortion is practiced occasionally as well as feticide, which is usually brought about by blows, compression, and external violence. Infanticide is extremely rare, as the mothers have a tradition that the next child will be blind.

" The Ainos live as nearly as possible in a state of nature. They have little or no ceremony at child-birth; before labor, the mother pursues her ordinary avocations as long as she can; after it is over, she considers it her duty to resume her work as soon as possible. The father and the friends often imbibe of rice *saké* too freely. I have learned of no religious or superstitious ceremony."

KALMUCKS.

The Kalmucks, the most numerous of all the Mongolian people, may well serve as a type of the natural Mongolian, as they are nomads, without a fixed home, roaming over mountain and plain, unaffected by civilization; whether belonging to Europe or Asia, they inhabit only the most remote and inaccessible parts of either country, and yet they are far in advance of the nomads of the far north. For their medical knowledge the Kalmucks are indebted to the Buddhists, to the schools of Thibet, founded for the Lamas; among them medicine is a divine knowledge, and possesses its especial idol, Burchan. For the following excellent description of their obstetric customs I am indebted to Dr. Rudolph Krebel's work: Volksmedizin und Volksmittel verschiedener Völkerstämme Russlands. (Leipzig & Heidelberg. 1858.)

" As soon as labor begins, the friends of the patient assemble; their idol is brought forth, conspicuously placed above the sufferer's couch, and illuminated with a lamp. The parturient now takes to her bed in expectation of the coming pains, during which she squats, her buttocks resting upon her heels, grasping with her hands a pole, which is firmly attached to the chimney, and of sufficient length to afford her a comfortable support; behind her sits another woman, who compresses her body with both arms; but, if in better circumstances, the husband takes some vigorous young fellow into his 'kibitke,' who, after being hospitably treated, takes his seat on the floor, with the parturient on his knees, and with his arms encircling her body, he compresses the abdomen and with the palms of his hands rubs the uterine surface, being careful to stroke it from above downward, and to exercise compression in the same direction. As soon as the female attendant observes the appearance of the head in the vulva, she signals the crowd of men who have been waiting outside, who simultaneously fire their guns, in order to assist nature by the sudden fright which this will cause the patient. The poor either buckle broad leather belts around the abdomen of the patient as soon as labor begins, and try to hasten matters by pressure from above downward, or they press a cloth firmly over mouth and nose of the woman to try the effect of choking, so that the exertions of the struggling sufferer may possibly expel the tardy fetus.

" It is said that in difficult cases female assistants have for ages practiced version, and physicians among the Songars have performed embryotomy with the knife. We hardly need mention that superstitions play an important part in their management of labor.

" The young mother is looked upon as unclean for three weeks after confinement; she is never abed at any time over seven days during the puerperal state. Immediately after delivery mutton is given the patient, but only a little at a time, whilst broth is given in considerable quantities ; the amount of meat used is gradually increased.

" As soon as the child is born, the cord is tied and cut, and the placenta buried at a considerable depth within the ' kibitke.' The child is washed in salt water and wrapped in furs. The remnant of the cord is carefully preserved, and kept as a charm, considered especially valuable in their petty lawsuits. Until the remnant of the cord separates from the child, the father does not permit fire from the hearth to be taken from his hut. The wealthy sometimes keep a wet nurse ; the poor nurse their own children, not unfrequently up to the very time when prevented by a succeeding pregnancy. Additional nourishment is given the child during the first year. During the first days the infant is not given the breast, but a piece of raw mutton tallow to suckle. The mortality is great among children, especially during the second year, on account of coarse food and hereditary syphilis."

NEGROES.

LOANGO-NEGROES.

I have chosen the Bafiotos, or negroes of Loango—a people of Central Africa—as representatives of the Blacks, as they are a fair type, somewhat above the majority of their neighbors; and because I am enabled to follow closely the excellent description of their traditions and customs by Dr. Peschuel-Loesche in the Zeitschrift fuer Ethnologie for 1878 (Inidiscretes aus Loango, p. 17). Menstruation seems to begin with the thirteenth, more rarely the twelfth year, and the cleanliness of the people does not permit an interruption of the daily bath, even during the continuance of the monthly flow. The idea of uncleanliness during the period, and during child-bed, prevails among the Loango women, as among most of their neighbors; and while menstruating a female must not approach or enter the huts of men. Woman, among the Loangos, ranks higher than among most African tribes, and instead of the long, pendent, breast which the negroes ordinarily cultivate, the Bafioto woman prides herself upon a firm mamma, and binds or straps the breast in case it threatens to drag; hence a Loango woman does not develop a long breast, and is never seen, like many of her black sisters, carrying on her back a suckling child, which is nursing the breast thrown over the shoulder.

They are a moral people; religious ceremonies, continuing many days, accompany the appearance of menstruation in the girl; for days she is isolated; strict laws govern the act of cohabitation, and the seduction of a maiden is looked upon as a misfortune which has befallen the entire land. They delight in children; hence abortion, as may be supposed, rarely occurs among this people, although sometimes practiced by elderly females of immoral character, who dread confinement; and they effect it by eating freely of red pepper, and by kneading and compressing the abdomen.

Twins and triplets are not killed; deformed children are quickly put aside; such as have only slight deformities are sometimes permitted to live; but even a mother's love cannot save them in case that popular feeling should be such as to consider them, for some reason or other, as possessed of any witchcraft.

It depends merely upon an accidental combination of circumstances whether an ill-formed child is doomed as a "ndodschi" (deformed bearer of misfortune), or simply as a "muana-mu-bi" (ugly, bad child); no fault is found with the mother. This superstition may go so far as to accuse a still unborn child; the mother is then given a poison bark, which is used in the official test ordeals, in the firm belief that the "ndodschi," if such a one exists, will be rendered harmless by being aborted—in case the mother should die in the ordeal her guilt is thus proven.

The pregnant woman is not forbidden to cohabit; she avoids garments of a red color, wearing white or blue, or simple native bark-fiber; she drinks no more rum lest the child should be marked, but this superstition is rapidly losing ground.[1] Charms favorable to women are erected in the hut, and worn upon the body—wise women, "ngangas" and neighbors are of course consulted.

The act of parturition is not difficult as a rule, and within a few hours the mother is enabled to again take up her accustomed work.. Skilled assistance of any kind is unknown—men are not permitted to be about. In difficult cases the neighboring huts, with a feeling of delicacy, are cleared; the children sent out of the village, and the assistants raise their voices in order to drown the lamentations of the patient in the general noise. Confinement takes place whilst the patient is standing, leaning against the wall, or kneeling, inclined forward, resting upon her arms, because the desired head-presentation is supposed to come about most readily in this position. The child is caught upon a bit of cloth or matting, that it may not touch the ground. If labor is retarded, the patient seeks her couch, casts herself down prone upon her stomach, and thus seeks to further labor by mechanical pressure. If expulsion is not furthered by these means, the assembled

---

[1] Evidently a very decided proof of advancing civilization.

women take charge of the case, especially if a primipara; arms and legs are seized, whilst some old woman, who squats down, takes the head of the patient upon her lap, presses a gag firmly upon mouth and nose in order to choke the sufferer, so that finally the child is forced out amid the spasmodic convulsions that follow. These means rarely fail—better ones at least are not known. Rupture of the perineum is not unfrequent. If a woman is overtaken with labor pains away from friends and help, she prevents at least that the child should fall to the ground and carries it home well covered.

The placenta is wrapt up and buried—secrecy of their labors seems to be entirely due to the prevalent feeling of modesty. The navel string is measured off to the double length of the first joint of the thumb, or to the knee, and is then cut, not with a knife, but with a sharp edge of a leaf-stalk of the bil palm. The assistants then seat themselves about a fire which has been lighted in the hut, and pass the new born babe from lap to lap, whilst with well-warmed hands the navel string is compressed and its drying off thus greatly hastened. This object is attained within twenty-four hours ; the parched and deadened remnant is thrust off with the thumb nail and cast into the fire, lest it should become food for the rats. If this should be devoured by them the child grows up wicked. Until the cord has been separated from the body and has been burnt, no male, not even the father, is admitted to the hut.

During the first days the child is not given the breast— the qualities of the colostrum seem recognized ; at least this is called "tschida fuenna," and the milk later "tschiali." In order to further the flow of milk the young mother drinks hot water for many months, and washes herself with a decoction of the leaf of the castor-bean plant. The genitals are cleansed and rubbed with bunches of these same leaves, well soaked in water, until all secretions cease.

The young mother takes frequent baths in some secluded spot, not too far from her hut; she seats herself in a slight excavation in the ground, which has been lined with mats, and whilst her assistants or friends are pouring hot and cold water alternately over her body, she is thoroughly kneaded and rubbed—massage. The child, especially in case that it should perspire, is bathed several times a day in cold water, into which charms have been dipped. The new born child remains within the hut for two or four months. The father and other men can only see it after the navel string has separated from the body, and even then only if they have not cohabited during the preceding night. The negroes themselves assign the suspicion of their wives as a reason for this exclusion, because they wish to retain control of them and prevent them from becoming dissolute, as mothers are prohibited from sexual intercourse during the period of lactation. This period averages twelve or fourteen months, but varies greatly, as some wean their children when the first teeth appear; others when they begin to talk. No Loango mother trusts her child to the care of another; they nurse the child just as civilized mothers do; they even hold down the breast with the fingers in the same manner. The breast is only given at certain times, no other food being offered in the intervals. The child seizes a part of the areola in addition to the entire nipple.

During the first months, while the child is carefully confined to the hut in which it was born, the mother goes out at will attending to her duties; but the homes of the men she dare not enter, not even that of her husband, whose visits she, however, receives, as the father loves to fondle his baby; later, the mother carries her baby in a cloth tied to her back, and even sometimes quite a large child is carried astraddle of her hips, a position in which the father is proud to carry about even his good-sized offspring. The Loango mother is very fond of her child, and it is no wonder, when we consider the attractive, oddly humorous, jolly appearance of the little negroes. Whilst the children are confined to the hut, two names are given them—a boy is called Nsau (elephant), a girl, Mputa (lovey, chickey). Their first appearance outside of the hut gives rise to a holiday; the mother, in festive garments, receives the villagers and their congratulations, whilst seated in front of her hut with her child upon her arms. A name is given the new-comer with a kind of baptism by some relative, usually the uncle, and, if we may so express it, citizenship is thereby extended to him.

THE RED RACES.

Primitive customs among our North American Indians are rapidly disappearing. As the war-bonnet of eagle plumes has given way to the unromantic felt hat—the tomahawk and bow and arrow to the revolver and breech-loading rifle—so are the original obstetric customs, traditionary among the red people for ages, yielding to the influence of civilization: the few warlike tribes, who still retain the ways of their ancestors, are rapidly dying out; those who have quietly settled down upon the reservation are accepting the habits of the whites, and their parturient squaws are delivered as they have been taught by the agency-physician or the army-surgeon; in fact, primitive obstetric customs are so speedily passing away that more than one of the agency-physicians answered with some surprise to the circular, kindly sent among them, for me, by the Smithsonian Institute, that he had observed nothing peculiar; that the squaws of the tribe were delivered on the back, and their habits were the same as those of their white sisters. Many of the tribes, nevertheless, still retain their peculiar customs, but all of my informants unite in the statement that it is very difficult to obtain any information from them upon these points. It is rare that men are permitted to witness, or even be near a labor scene; and white physicians are not called in unless it be a desperate case. Indians are moreover very reticent upon this point and very unwilling to impart any information regarding their women or the functions peculiar to them;

this is strange, too, as they are by no means a modest people.

There are many points of resemblance in the obstetric customs of the various Indian tribes, and in many features

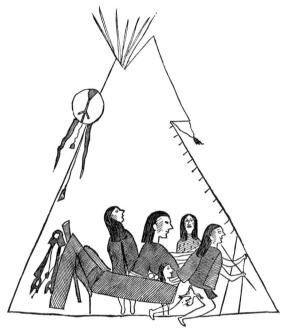

FIG. 54—Kiowa Labor.

they differ. The kneeling posture, for instance, is the one most commonly assumed by the squaw in labor, and yet among certain tribes almost all the other positions can be found, though rarely that upon the lap of the husband; this is a trouble and indignity which the laziness and pride of the Indian-brave will not submit to.

As I cannot detail the customs of the various tribes, I will confine myself to the obstetric practice of the Indians of the northwest, and of the more easterly prairie tribes. As regards the former I shall accept the statement of Dr. John Field, of Sheridan, Oregon, who has given the following very interesting account of his long stay among the tribes, especially while physician to the Grand Ronde Agency in Oregon; he says:

The Indians of the Pacific Coast.

Women belonging to the Indian tribes on the northwest coast are attended in labor by a number of older squaws, as many as may be necessary. These attendants are not especially skilled midwives, but the mothers, if living near enough, or some other older friend and a few of the neighbors. It is among these people as it is among the whites, there is always some old woman in every tribe, band or settlement, who is looked upon as an authority in these cases, who is considered an expert manipulator and whose every order or suggestion is implicitly obeyed.

During the first stage of labor, the patient will usually keep on her feet, moving about the lodge, or now and then lying on her bed for a short period at a time. At the recurrence of each pain the parturient will frequently utter a plaintive cry. In this she differs somewhat from her white sister, who will most generally announce the occurrence of pain by a sound which has, by the old women, been determined "grunt," "grunting;" the former gives vent to a low, plaintive cry, which the word "wail" or "whine" seems to express more nearly than any other. When the parturient lies down she usually reclines upon her back, with the legs semi-flexed upon the thighs, the thighs likewise flexed upon the body.

No assistance is rendered at the time of a pain during the first stage, but the attendants are all ready, and willing to help when the proper time comes.

The patient takes to her bed and lies on her back—her head slighly elevated. This bed or pallet is universally on the floor, and near the fire if the weather is cold. Her legs are well flexed upon her thighs, and her thighs upon her abdomen; knees and feet are each supported by an assistant; she herself usually uses her hand to press against her thighs, or when the pains become severe, to compress her own abdomen over the fundus uteri.

The officiating accoucheur—if the term is allowable—crouches upon the pallet at the feet of the parturient, with her hands pressed upon the nates, perineum vulva or abdomen of patient, as circumstances in her judgment may require.

She does not rely upon vaginal examination, nor indeed does she at all practice that means either of diagnosis or assistance to her patient.

As the case progresses, and the expulsive pains increase in severity, the abdomen of the parturient is firmly compressed over the fundus uteri by the hands of an assistant. She now uses her own hands to press upon her thighs, and does not pull at the hands of an attendant as so many white women do.

The abdominal manipulations before referred to are practiced by an assistant, kneeling by the side of the patient, with her face towards the patient's feet. She spreads her fingers in such a manner as to grasp the entire fundus uteri as nearly as possible. When the uterus is being contracted by the force of nature the assistant follows the fundus with her hands, firmly grasping the organ, and gently but firmly pressing downward. When the pain subsides, she still keeps her firm hold of the uterus, and does not allow it to relax, at least she does all she can to prevent this.

If the case is a tedious one, and the head is slow to pass, another method is resorted to in addition to the one mentioned.

The woman is seized by two attendants, who grasp her around the thorax, immediately under the arms, raise her body off the bed, and support her in an erect position, so far as her body is concerned. She is permitted to rest upon her knees or feet, according to the peculiar notion of the accoucheuse, or according to attending circumstances.

By these means, and in the position above mentioned, she is as firmly supported as is possible for the attendants to do.

The abdominal pressure is firmly kept up until the end of the labor.

The accompanying illustration, although a labor scene among the Mexican Indians in the vicinity of San Luis

Potosi, and there photographed for me by Dr. G. Barroeta, so well represents the relative position of patient and assistants, as here described, that I have inserted it.

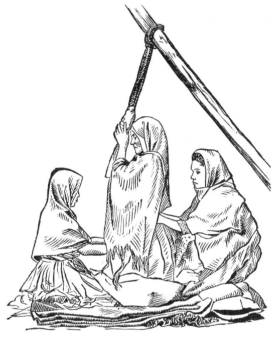

FIG. 55.—Mexican Indians.

Towards the close, and while the woman is in the position last named, the accoucheuse remains crouched at the feet of the parturient, supporting the perineum and vulva with the palms of her hands. As soon as the head emerges fully through the vulva, the accoucheuse takes it between her hands and makes traction so that the shoulders and. body of the child will be the more speedily delivered.

The child is received into the lap of the accoucheuse whether the mother is in the erect position or lying down.

The umbilical cord is tied and divided in a few moments after delivery, and the child is laid to one side out of the way. The delivery of the placenta is expected at once after the birth of the child and without further trouble; in order to facilitate speedy expulsion the accoucheuse and assistants resort to certain manipulations.

This effort to assist the uterus in casting off the placenta is made immediately after the child is born, and stowed away in a safe place.

If the case has been an easy one, and the woman has not been raised from her couch, the first efforts to obtain the placenta are made as she lies there, the accoucheuse, making gentle but tolerable firm traction on the cord with one hand, manipulates the uterine globe with the other. At the same time, if thought necessary, an assistant will press (by spreading the fingers of both hands) and even kneed the abdomen, with the view of pressing the secundines out of the uterine cavity. If these efforts fail while the woman is in the recumbent posture, she is raised to the erect position, and thus supported, as in cases of difficult delivery of the child. The uterine globe is then firmly pressed and kneeded, whilst the accoucheuse makes more or less firm traction upon the cord.

But if the case should be one of abnormal attachment, or hour-glass contraction, they know no method of procedure that promises success. Frequently the patient will survive, escaping blood poisoning, and the secundines will be cast off in a state of disorganization.

By making persistent inquiries I learn that they seldom fail in sufficiently stimulating the uterus to cast off the placenta.

AFTER TREATMENT.

The treatment resorted to after delivery is not alike among all tribes. Some, with whom I have come in contact, require the puerpera to keep up on her feet during the greater part of the day—taking short walks about the camp, resting when weariness becomes oppressive; while walking she uses a staff, for the double purpose of support while upon her feet, and also as an instrument of relief; as she slowly steps about the body is frequently bent forward, bringing the abdominal walls immediately over the uterus against the upper end of the staff, while the hand of the woman is upon the end of the stick in the same way as that of a man walking with a cane.

This practice is kept up for a period of three or four days, when the puerpera is thought to be well; the prescribed walks varying with periods of rest upon her couch.

The object—as I am informed by the old women of the tribe—is to facilitate the flow of the lochia.

They know that a certain amount of blood should escape, and think that if the patient should lie down in bed this would accumulate in the abdominal cavity, and cause death. From all I can learn, by inquiries of those of the tribes who are old enough to remember the practice among the Indians in this region before the time that the white man came among them, this procedure in the after-treatment was solely for the purpose of encouraging a free flow of the lochia, and I further learn that no case of death from hemorrhage had then been known to occur.

Some of the Indian tribes in this country follow a different course of after-treatment.

As soon as possible after delivery the puerpera is placed on a bed on the floor of the lodge, and securely wrapped in blankets, or whatever kind of covering they have. The bed is placed near the fire, if the weather is cool, and she is kept in this closely wrapped condition. When asking for an explanation of this method of treating their lying-in women, I was told that it was to keep the patient from taking cold, and having fever (somewhat like the Siamese). In this condition she is kept for the period of four or five days, except such times as she is compelled to attend the calls of nature. When freed from this restriction, she at once resumes the care of the babe as well as the duties naturally falling to the lot of an Indian squaw.

During the period that I was living among these Indians —two and one-half years—I neither saw or heard of a case of puerperal fever, eclampsia, or any other diseases peculiar to the lying-in woman. Neither did a death during confinement come under my immediate observation, and but few Indian women have any mammary trouble after their confinement, notwithstanding the fact that they are exposed to the same cause that is a prolific source of such complications among whites.

EASTERN TRIBES.

As it is impossible for me to make use of all of the extremely valuable and interesting information received by kindly responses from the surgeons of the army and agencies among the various Indian tribes, I will close with a description of the obstetric customs among the more easterly tribes, the Cheyennes, Arapahoes, Kiowas, Comanches, and eastern Apaches, given me by Maj. W. H. Forwood, U. S. A., now stationed at Fort Omaha, Nebraska. Maj. Forwood resided for over five years among these tribes, who are scattered over the plains of Kansas, Nebraska, Colorado and the Indian Territory, and constantly came in contact with them at Forts Larned and Sill, where they congregated and frequently applied for treatment. He says:

" The customs prevailing among the above named tribes are similar, and the following instance may well characterize them :

" In August, 1869, at Fort Sill, I. T., I was called upon by a few men and squaws of the Comanche tribe for the purpose of securing my services in the case of a patient who had born two children, and had had difficulty at both of her confinements. They anticipated difficulty again, and this was the reason for summoning me, which otherwise would not have been considered necessary. At the proper time I rode to the encampment on Cache Creek, a few miles from the Post, where I found the lodges pitched in a wide circuit on high open ground, near the stream. A short distance outside the camp, and in rear of the patient's family lodge, were arranged the accommodations for the confinement. A shelter had been constructed of green boughs six or seven feet high, by setting up brush or bushes, with the leaves on, around the circumference of a circle, about eight feet in diameter. An entrance was provided by breaking the circle and overlapping the two unjoined ends. In a line outside the entrance were three stakes, ten paces apart, set firmly upright in the ground, four feet high, made from the stems of small saplings with the bark left on.

" Inside of this shelter were two holes for the reception of fluids of any kind and the steaming of the parts, and stakes for the support of the parturient. Three stakes were also planted outside of this enclosure, so that the patient, when surprised by a pain, as she walks about in the intervals, may at once kneel down and find a support. (See Fig. 13, and for full description p. 35. Posture.) So my patient was walking about with her assistant, a female relative, and as each pain came on she knelt down, grasping a stake, whilst the assistant, standing or kneeling behind her, seized her about the waist and kneaded and compressed the abdomen.

" She was a full Comanche squaw, aged about 20, of slight frame, in good general health; had given birth to two healthy children, but had suffered tedious labor with both, and some delay in the discharge of the placenta. Her dress consisted of a body, a skirt, and two leg pieces made of deer skin, and nicely ornamented with beads, silver shells, etc. The body was of one skin, with a hole in the middle for the head, the ends coming down in front and rear, fastened at the sides under the arms, making a sort of flowing sleeve, and reaching below the waist. The skirt piece was of about two skins, merely wound around, extending a little below the knees, and secured by a leather belt at the waist. The leggings were separate pieces, with moccasins attached, extending above the knees, fastened by a narrow strip at the outside to the waist-belt, colored, fringed and ornamented at the leg; flowing hair, beads at the neck, and a number of brass rings about the wrists.

" Examination, to which she had submitted with evident disgust and not without some persuasion, revealed the membranes ruptured, waters escaped, parts rather dry, but head presenting favorably, and pains moderately strong, so that the labor was deemed practical within a reasonable time by the efforts of nature. Without making any suggestions or offering further interference, I sat down to "make medicine," as they thought, but in reality to improve the opportunity for observation. The patient was assisted by a woman of middle age and some experience in such cases, while a considerable number of other squaws of all ages thronged around, making suggestions, talking, singing, groaning and gesticulating, but no men came near.

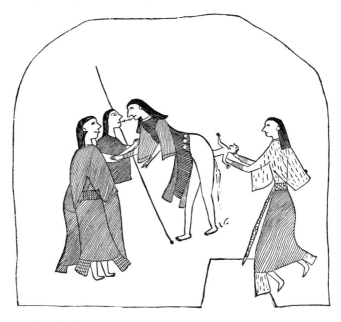

FIG. 56.—Kiowa midwife blowing an emetic into patient's mouth.

" She never assumed the recumbent position, nor did the assistant make any attempt at vaginal examination. There was no great effort on her part to restrain the feelings or submit patiently to suffering, and the throng of women inside and out kept up a continual noise and clatter. Meantime the chief medicine man of the tribe in a neighboring lodge was making strenuous exertions to help the patient by means which I was not permitted to see, but which could be plainly heard going on incessantly. The ceremony was performed alone in a closed lodge, with fire, and consisted, so far as I knew, in drumming, singing, shouting, dancing, running round the fire, jumping over it, manœuvring with knives, and the like antics. Medicine making of this sort is very common among the Indians, and is always conducted with great solemnity and seriousness, and with full faith in its effect. The rationale is based on the idea that disease is an evil spirit entering the patient, and must by some magic influence be coaxed, scared or driven out. The internal administration of medicine, excepting emetics, is seldom practiced, and emetics are scrupulously avoided in cases of labor, owing to the direction in which they act. But in the midst of a vast amount of sheer nonsense they possess some good practical ideas, such as the buffalo hair pessary worn with benefit by many women, the hot stone in labor, which is sometimes modified into a steam bath by covering the shelter tightly with skins and pouring water on the stone. At a former confinement of the patient, a practical application had been made of the effect of fear in routing the child from its lodging place. She was brought out on the plain, and Eissehaby, a noted chief, mounted on his swiftest steed, with all his war paint and equipments on, charged down upon her at full speed, turning aside only at the last moment, when she expected to be pierced through the body and trampled under foot. This is said to have caused an immediate expulsion of the child.

"As the crisis was evidently approaching, another examination was made, with the patient on her back on a robe, and the child was soon born, the placenta following a few moments later. Immediately the greatest excitement prevailed, the monotonous songs and doleful cries were changed to sounds of rejoicing, and the noise and din were louder than ever, but of a far more pleasant character. The moment the placenta escaped the patient sprang up, buckled on a stout leather belt, mingled with the crowd and soon disappeared, without apparently taking the slightest notice of her child. I took up the baby and offered it to some of the bystanders, but each one shrank back and would not even touch it. Presently a woman, whom I had not seen before, appeared and took charge of it. She was assigned to the duty of receiving and having the little stranger initiated into the world with proper ceremony. This, in case of a boy, would probably be some simple little nonsense performed by an old chief, and in case of a girl, by the squaw herself.

"An instance came under my notice once in which an imaginary object (a ball it was said to be) was blown into the mouth and placed down in the ribs somewhere about the heart, where it was to remain, the supposed effect being to give courage and protect against harm. The medicine chief approached, and placing his two hands in front of his chest and throat, made a gulping effort as though bringing something up out of his own body, leaned over and blew quickly into the patient's mouth, and the thing was done.

"The Indians tie the cord with one ligature and cut it almost a foot from the child's body. The placenta is then secretly and mysteriously disposed of in various ways not unlike those often practiced by old women among ourselves. Their resources in case of retained placenta, so far as I know, are limited to forcible compression of the abdomen, traction upon the cord, and efforts to reach it with the hand in the vagina, in which the patient as well as the assistant take part. They never neglect to pay the doctor his fee, lest he should become angry, and, by the power of his arts, bring some calamity upon the patient in future, and that ceremony was not overlooked in this instance. I was brought to the chief's lodge and formally presented with a pony of my own selection, but, as they feared the poor creature would be very lonely away from its companions, I was requested to let it run with the herd, and consider it mine—with the herd of course it remained."

A surgeon who has been stationed for some years at Camp Sheridan, in the Spotted Tail Indian Agency, in the midst of from seven to twelve thousand Sioux Indians, principally of the great Brulé branch of the nation, and who has carefully inquired into their customs, writes : " My inquiries into their obstetric habits were attended with difficulties, as these Indians, never talkative, become quite reticent as soon as any questions are asked concerning their peculiarities. No very definite custom or practice seems to be followed; the most common is, that several matrons preside as midwives in the lodge of the parturient, which is, especially in delayed cases, filled to suffocation with indifferently solicitous (?) relations and friends.

"During the first stage the squaw sits or lies about grunting vociferously, but during the expulsion of the fetus her posture is erect, or nearly so, with her arms around the neck of a stout male support, mostly a young bachelor buck. The child is received by the attendant squaw, and the placenta promptly follows, as a rule. She is then put to bed, and the lochia received on old clothes, which are burned.

"These Indians, though nearly regardless of what we consider as modesty with regard to defecation and urination, are quite superstitious about the functions peculiar to women. On the first menstruation of a maiden quite a ceremonious feast is held, at which the relatives and attending friends congratulate the maiden, and her parents, on the dawn of her womanhood, for she is now a woman. During the whole of each menstrual period (or "moon in the ass," as they term it) the female is hedged about with restrictions. She is considered unclean, must refrain from certain things, and is disqualified from assisting or participating in any of the ceremonies of her tribe.

"Other of their customs, also, are quite peculiar. The female stands to urinate and sits during defecation, whilst the male sits on his haunches to urinate, and stands during defecation; the male mounts his horse from the right side, the female from the left."

Among the Indians of Montana the usual name for a child for the first year or two, before a permanent name is bought of the medicine man, is " Mai, Tsä Barkea-Tsä-careash," which is a word applied to a spirit, and also to the gray-crowned finch (Leucosticte tephrocotis), into which bird young children are believed to enter on their death.

Twins cause their parents to be greatly envied ; but if a squaw becomes pregnant while still nursing, the child at the breast is said to die in four cases out of five from diarrhea and marasmus.

Among the Modocs and Klamaths, the husband refrains from eating all flesh of fish or game for five days after the birth of a child, and the mother refrains from the same for ten days. At each menstrual period the woman refrains from flesh for five days and is more or less isolated from the male portion of the family, the same custom prevailing after an abortion.

These five and ten days periods are the same I have repeatedly spoken of among the natives of India and Africa.

Certain of the tribes demand that the father take to the woods and absent himself for some days from the family lodge and the encampment, and if it be his first child he caches himself until the child is a week old.

It is only the young men who practice this, as they are so ashamed of the occurrence.

At the end of this time, or as soon as the father is able, he calls all his relations and friends together and has a feast of boiled dog—provided the child be a male.

Much of this information, especially the last, regarding the O-g-a-l-la-l-la Sioux, comes from the well known Indian Scout, Will. E. Everett.

Although I should like to enter more fully into the customs of the various Indian tribes, the above will suffice to show the intimate relation between the obstetric customs among the yellow, black and red races.

I have made use of the last three illustrations, although not bearing directly upon the customs of the tribes here referred to, on account of their extreme interest.

Figures 54 and 56 I obtained through the kindness of Capt. M. Barber, surgeon U. S. A., of Fort Sill, who had them made by a Kiowa artist to illustrate the customs of his people.

Fig. 54 represents a labor scene in a Kiowa *tepee.* The

patient is on her knees, grasping a tent pole fastened at right angles to two upright ones ; one assistant is kneading her back, whilst another is attending to the child which is in the act of being born. A gun, saddle and "G" string, the peculiar articles of male apparel, are hung at the head of the couch to induce the birth of a boy.

Fig. 56 represents the midwife blowing something into the patient's mouth to make her vomit and strain, and thus assist the labor pains. She here rests herself upon the pole, which plays so important a role in their labors, sometimes serving as a support to the kneeling patient (fig. 54), sometimes as a means of expression when she leans upon it with her stomach. This scene is represented taking place in the "medicine lodge"—why, Dr. Barber could not inform me.

Fig. 55 is taken from a photograph secured for me by my friend Dr. G. Barroeta, of San Louis Potosi, Mexico, and well illustrates the posture of patient and assistants as assumed in labor by the Indians of that region. I have in an earlier chapter described the scene more in detail and pictured it so as to show the position of the assistant's hands ; here they are concealed, as is customary, beneath the clothing, so as not to expose the person of the patient.